INVISIBLE ILLNESS

SILENT SUFFERING

Understanding the physical,
emotional, and spiritual effects

of Fibromyalgia

Patrice Burke M.A.
and
Diana Hahlbohm

FORWARD

Every day thousands of people suffer from the devastating effects of illnesses that are not visible to others. Because they appear to be healthy, without any physical limitations, they are often misunderstood, sometimes thought to be lazy or a hypochondriac. Many suffer alone, without the support of family and friends because they don't know how to express their needs or explain their challenges. I live with the ongoing challenges of Fibromyalgia, and at one time Chronic Fatigue Syndrome. Fibromyalgia is a muscle disorder, or for the sake of this book, an illness, that is not visible to others. As a matter of fact, if you were to meet me at most any given moment, you would never know that I live with this chronic illness that has negatively impacted almost every area of my life. And so it is with so many others who live with a chronic illness that is not visible to those around them and to those to whom they would normally look to for support. I decided to write this book about my own personal journey with Fibromyalgia, so that others who share similar struggles would have someone to identify with and validate their struggles. And perhaps, to also help those with friends and/or relatives that have such a chronic illness, better understand the challenges that face the one they care about.

I will not go into a lot of medical aspects of Chronic Fatigue Syndrome and Fibromyalgia. As a matter of fact, my focus will be on Fibromyalgia as this is the ongoing illness that I live with and that so many others live with. What I will focus on is the impact that Fibromyalgia has had on the emotional, social, spiritual, and economical aspects of my life. Since the

Christian faith has played an integral part in my life, I will also explore how my faith has helped determine how I have faced the challenges presented by living with Fibromyalgia.

After most chapters my close friend, and fellow sufferer of Fibromyalgia, will speak about her experience with both CFS and Fibromyalgia. Diana has dealt with these illnesses for much longer than I have, and more intensely. I believe her story will greatly enhance one's understanding of the devastating effects of this illness. In addition, Diana is married and can shed some light on how the symptoms of Fibromyalgia can create challenges in a marriage.

My prayer is that if you live with Fibromyalgia or other such illness, that this book will bring you understanding and validation around the many challenges that you face each day. Also, that it will help you find ways to express your needs and challenges to others, perhaps, by letting them read my story if you find yours too difficult to tell. Most of all, I pray it will bring you Hope. Hope that you can have life worth living. Hope that your life can indeed be filled with peace and joy.

ACKNOWLEDGEMENTS

We would like to give a special thanks those who have supported us in writing this book, through much prayer and devoted friendship over the years. In the times when Fibromyalgia was unknown to most of the world, my mother, Janet Bohanon, taught me to seek out knowledge in order to be empowered for the long, hard, and sometimes dark journey ahead. As I watched her pray and seek help and guidance from above, I was inspired by how she instantly began to help others with chronic illness. God has been the main source of our inspiration and to Him we give all our praise.

We would like to extend a special heartfelt "thank you" to Diana's husband, Danny Hahlbohm, for the beautiful artwork on the cover of this book and for all his help in the creative process to make this book possible. Without his knowledge and help, this book might not have come into fruition.

Danny has been instrumental in spreading the Word of God through his art ministry for the last 40 years. You can see all of Danny's artwork at his website: www.inspired-art.com

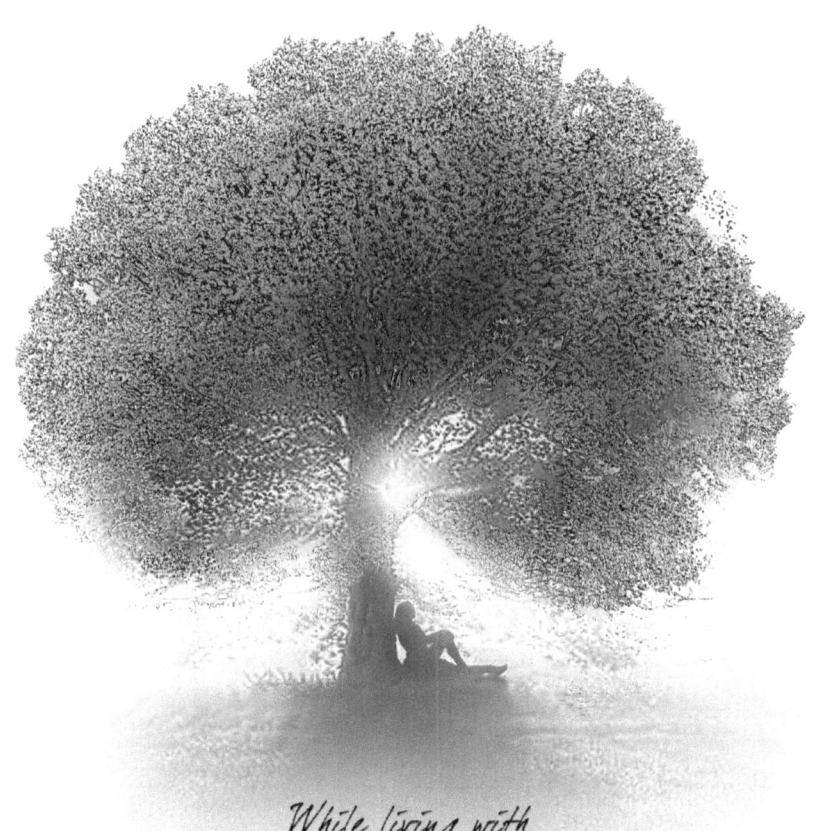

While living with
ongoing chronic pain and
fatigue, I often felt like Fibromyalgia
was draining the life out of me. And so,
I would go outside and sit under this huge
green tree and imagine it was the tree of life, so
strong, so full of energy, healing my body and soul.

TABLE OF CONTENTS

Printed in the United States of America.
© 2017 Patrice Burke and Diana Hahlbohm

Website: www.inspired-art.com
www.lightofeden.com

Email: fibropd@yahoo.com
Patriceburke50@yahoo.com
Hahlbohmd@yahoo.com

Unless otherwise noted, all scripture quotations are from the KING JAMES VERSION (KJV): public domain.

Scripture quotations marked (NIV) are taken from the THE HOLY BIBLE, NEW INTERNATIONAL VERSION ®. Copyright© 1973, 1978, 1984, 2011 by Biblica, Inc.TM. Used by permission of Zondervan.

CHAPTER 1

WELCOME TO MY WORLD

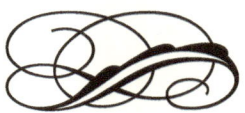

It is morning, time to get out of bed and join the land of the living. At least that is what I tell myself. My body feels stiff, my joints hurt and I feel this dull ache all over. I often feel like there is this dark cloud just hanging over my bed, giving me a sense of doom along with a strong desire to stay put. Even though I went to bed at a reasonable time, I simply feel exhausted. When the pain and fatigue are at their worst, my mind can go into dark places, like thinking life is not worth living and wishing I had not woken up. This may be tough to hear, but it is a reality, one I deal with on a regular basis. So, I push aside all the doom and gloom thoughts and purposely and willfully grasp on to ones that are life giving, rather than sucking the life out of me. For me, it is my faith in a good and kind God. I turn my thoughts to Him and ask for help. After I do this, I have a little chat with myself before my feet even hit the ground. I remind myself that the flare-ups don't last forever, that God is in control of my life not me, and I remind myself of how much I enjoy living. Now I can start my day, difficult as it might be.

Welcome to my world. A world touched by chronic illness, Fibromyalgia to be more specific. And this is only the beginning. All day, every day is touched by this illness. What is it? Well, I am not sure even the doctors really know. Right now the general consensus is that it is the result of over active nerve cells in the muscles. When you say it, it actually doesn't sound all that bad. And most people with this illness look healthy. Most commercials around this illness make it appear that Fibromyalgia is just a case of aching muscles. Although one commercial does mention how it interferes with one's life. Still, the depth of suffering that this illness can bring into one's life is truly not understood by most people. The result of this inability to see evidence of the illness often results in those with Fibromyalgia being considered lazy and/or hypochondriacs. So, let's take a look at just what this illness entails and how it can impact a person's life.

Diana Speaks:

As I read Patrice's introduction, there is comfort in knowing that someone else understands this illness as much as I do, if not more, and that by writing about our experience, we can share this journey with others. We hope that by doing so, we can help other people better understand their own challenges. We have found that one thing that often helps us feel better emotionally, is knowing that we are not alone and that someone understands this illness and is willing to share their struggles and victories with us. Fellowship and sharing with others can be a form of medication, helping to alleviate our pain. And so, we invite you, the reader, to join us on this journey because you are NOT alone.

My day begins before dawn as I awaken with a burning sensation in what feels like my whole body, inside and out. There is a pain I chase with medication, trying to stay one step ahead of it to keep myself from falling off the edge of sanity. So here I go, with my medication at my bedside as I reach for that source of help that is within my grasp. Then comes the waiting game as I anticipate some form of relief so that I can begin my brand new day. Before coffee, before my morning meditation with the Lord, I reach for pills because without some relief from this pain, I cannot begin fresh on a new day's journey. There are so many times during the morning when my husband will come to check on me and ask how I am doing. I usually say, " I am waiting for my pills to work". He knows what I mean. He is aware that I am in pain. It is difficult for him to bare the fact that I am in hurting, knowing that he cannot fix it, as many husbands would want to do.

Welcome to what sometimes feels like a powerless state; but in fact, there can be joy in the morning as I have faith in the treasures that will unfold. I try not to linger in the dark places because that makes me feel so much worse. I am not alone; there are an estimated 10 million people who suffer with this just in America alone. Patrice and I will share with you, from the perspective of just two of the 10 million, as we join together to shed light, share love and friendship with all who choose to come along on this quest with us.

CHAPTER 2

AND SO IT BEGINS

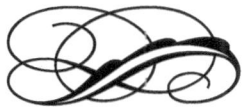

In 1986 I was a single mother of two working three part time jobs. One of those jobs was as an aerobics instructor. I actually felt and looked better than I ever had. What I did not know was that the stress of juggling motherhood and working three part-time jobs was creating a stress in my body that would make it vulnerable to a very strange and little known syndrome or virus called Chronic Fatigue Syndrome (CFS). Now many believe that CFS and Fibromyalgia are the same illness as they have many of the same symptoms. Others believe they are separate illnesses. I tend to believe the second school of thought. Most research around CFS indicates that it is a virus that attacks the immune system. I believe that Fibromyalgia is often a symptom of CFS.

During the autumn of 1986, I got the flu and it lasted for two weeks. I have never been so sick. It left me bound to my bed for almost the entire two weeks. This was unusual for me as I was rarely sick. Although my health would improve enough that I could go back to work, I never really fully recovered. One of my part-time jobs had been as an aerobics instructor and I remember that after having the flu, I could barely get through a normal routine without feeling fatigued and experiencing some muscle soreness. I clearly remember one day after teaching a class, standing against a wall and slowly sliding down it until I was sitting on the floor. And, I was crying because I felt so exhausted. My muscles began to ache all over, especially when I exerted myself in any way.

Within in a year or so of the onset of the fatigue I had to stop doing aerobics and had to give up one of my other jobs, waitressing, because I could not physically keep up with it. I also noticed that I was becoming anxious and a bit down because I always felt so tired. By the end of about two or three years, my life became somewhat limited. I remember that I was still able to work a part-time job in an office but that my social life had almost completely disappeared. I simply did not have enough energy to socialize. This was especially difficult for me as I really enjoyed going out or just socializing with my friends. During this time I also started having repeated sinus infections and was constantly on antibiotics. Meanwhile, my doctor could not figure out what was wrong with me.

After a few years of muscles pain, one doctor did diagnose me with Fibromyalgia. I remember that she found trigger points on my body that were consistent with Fibromyalgia, but since so little was known about it and because I had so many other symptoms not usually associated with it, she just wasn't sure. However, she told me to call her when I had a sudden onset of muscle pain. Well, that summer I took my children to a water park and we swam all day long. About 48 hours later, I could not get out of bed. When I called this doctor, she confirmed the diagnosis of Fibromyalgia but still thought something else was going on. She explained that people with Fibromyalgia often don't feel the pain from exerting their muscles until about 24 to 48 hours later, rarely immediately after. Now I at least had some validation and a partial diagnosis.

Over the next 5 years my health would slowly erode until I was housebound, too sick to leave my home. The symptoms were all over the place, fatigue being the most prominent one and muscle soreness running a close second. I can remember the fatigue being so severe that at one point I could only walk with someone helping me or leaning on something. And the pain was intolerable, especially when it radiated into my neck and face. Then there were those constant sinus infections. It seemed that no matter what I did or how many antibiotics I took they just kept coming back. I must say though, I never got the fevers that so many people with CFS got. Emotionally I was becoming more and more fragile. I started having nightmares at night, often waking up in a sweat with my heart pounding. There wasn't any one thing that I could remember that brought this on. I believe now it was a combination of not being able to work, worrying about taking care of my children, and concerns about just how sick I would get, that it just wreaked havoc on me emotionally.

Can you imagine being all alone with two children and having no income, unable to work, and barely being able to get out of bed? It all truly was one big nightmare.

Probably about three to four years into having CFS, after being housebound for about one year, this illness took on a new dimension. I started to have intense anxiety and panic attacks. It is believed by some, as I also believe, that the virus sometimes attacks the brain. You see, some people get CFS experiencing the fatigue and then get better in a few years. Others get it and experience more symptoms and recover over a period of time. Still others get all the neurological symptoms, like panic attacks, anxiety attacks, and even petit mall seizures, and either do not ever fully recover or recover to some degree after about seven years. Well, I got all the neurological symptoms and thought I just might be losing my mind. Fortunately, I found some articles on CFS and just knew that I had it. I then joined a CFS support group, which eventually led me to a Dr. Jay Krasner who, at the time, was familiar with this illness and how it presented. By the time I got to him, I had reached rock bottom. I could not leave my house, was having panic and anxiety attacks, periods of feeling like I was detached from my body, and had become so sensitive to my environment that I just stayed in my room all day. Then, I got the diagnosis. What a relief. I thought perhaps there was hope yet, and there was.

It took about seven years, but I did recover from CFS. It's hard to recall just how I recovered, but Dr. Krasner and I did work on getting the right combination of medications along with some natural supplements. It is different for everyone, but I remember that many of us in the support group did take some kind of an anti-depressant, which was important because when you struggle with a chronic illness, depression often sets in. Most of us also took at least the two natural supplements of Grape seed Extract and CQ10. But, as I said, each person was different.

I must say though, that all during my struggle with CFS, I attended a weekly church group that held me up in prayer. The leader of the group even gave me permission to call him when the anxiety got too intense or when I had nightmares. But I will get more into that when I talk about the different aspects of Fibromyalgia keeping in mind that many of the symptoms of Fibromyalgia that I will talk about also apply to CFS and other invisible illnesses.

So, while I did recover from CFS, the Fibromyalgia never really went away. It did, however, get better and stayed better for about seven years. Then, after several major surgeries it resurfaced and has been an active part of my life since. It is believed by many professionals that a chronic illness, ongoing untreated stress, and some emotional and/or physical trauma can make people susceptible to getting Fibromyalgia and can cause it to flare up once they have it. Now that I look back, I believe that both my stressful life style and getting CFS are root causes as to why I developed Fibromyalgia. And, I believe that when I underwent those two major surgeries, the trauma to my body caused the Fibromyalgia to become active after it had gotten better for those seven years.

So, now let's look at it more in depth and the different symptoms of Fibromyalgia, which keep in mind also presented in CFS, and how they might impact someone's life. Hopefully with better understanding of each symptom and how it can affect a person's life, person's struggling with Fibromyalgia, and/or another chronic illness, will be able to find more effective ways to cope with them. And, for those who know or live with people with Fibromyalgia, and/or other chronic illness, can better support them.

Diana Speaks:
I cannot begin my story without first mentioning my mother, Janet Bohanon, who along with myself and other family members came down with Mononucleosis in the 1970's from which none of us seemed to fully recover, which turned into CFS and Fibromyalgia. My mother and uncle were sicker than my brother and I, but none of us ever felt "normal" after this illness. It literally felt like we never bounced back as we continued to suffer with some fatigue and achy muscles. One doctor told my mother about something called the Epstein Barr Virus that attacked the immune system and often presented much like Mononucleosis. This virus could morph into a syndrome called Chronic Fatigue Syndrome (CFS). I don't know exactly the relation between all three of these illnesses, but when you see one, you need to consider the other. Anyway, my mother was relieved to finally have a name for what was attacking her body, Chronic Fatigue Syndrome and later diagnosed with Fibromyalgia. My uncle was also diagnosed with CFS. Since my brother and I had similar symptoms, we assumed, and correctly that

we also had CFS and Fibro.

Knowing that Chronic Fatigue Syndrome wasn't well known and that many people suffered with it, my mother felt that she could not just sit by and do nothing to help. She would go on to create the first National Chronic Fatigue Association. Her goal was to educate and equip others with the knowledge of this syndrome so that they could better help themselves and give more information family members. She began a newsletter from her small home in Kansas City with only 16 members and it would quickly grow to about 25,000 members and upward. Sadly, by the time the organization got to the 25,000 members, my mother was too weak to continue producing and mailing out that many newsletters by hand. Little did she know though, that one of those people that she had reached out to would use information in a newsletter to help get diagnosed with CFS and begin her road to understanding her illness better. This person was Patrice Burke, my friend from Massachusetts who I had yet to meet.

Skip forward now to Florida 2009 at a church luncheon, when Patrice sat across the table from me mentioned she had been struggling with a chronic illness for a long time. I asked her to explain and she began to tell her story. She talked about how it all began back in the mid 1980's and later talked about how a newsletter had helped her understand just what this illness was all about. I was shocked and amazed to find out that it was my mother's newsletter that helped Patrice to find the support and understanding she needed at one of the lowest physical and emotional points in her life. We both realized at that point that this surely was a "God thing", us meeting like that in a little church in Venice, Florida. We would go on to become dear friends. Since our earlier years when we were diagnosed with CFS, we both have gone on to be diagnosed with Fibromyalgia, as was my mother. So Fibromyalgia will be our focal point as this is the illness that continues to invade our lies. We do not want to stay isolated and imprisoned any longer. So, we break out of the box and fight to bring light to others as well.

It was clear that just like in the 1980's, God was working in our lives at specific times to bring us to one another in His divine and perfect timing. We are no longer observers, but companions seeking a way and means to help others, just like my mother did before me and whose example I want to follow, and so I carry on where she left off. Although much later than I would have liked, but still in time to care and share with one another and with you, the readers who now have come to join us.

I have struggled with chronic illness since my late teenage years. Simple tasks at times felt overwhelming. I remember so well when I was in my 20's and 30's, after becoming a wife and mother, raising three boys, what a struggle it was physically to be the interactive mother that I so wanted to be. During some of those years I lived across the alley from my mother and would walk over and help her organize and mail out all those newsletters that would go across the country. Who knows, I may have stamped and addressed one to Patrice.

I find that when I am in my worst pain that if I think about encouraging others with this illness, it actually disarms my powerless feeling and I am energized by love and compassion for others. I am reminded that my beloved mother made such a positive impact on others in her efforts to reach out and educate those with CFS and then Fibromyalgia. She was invited to the White House, by Barbara Bush to discuss this debilitating illness, which was such an honor. Even though my mother was to weak to go, it is a testament of how one person can create such a rippling effect through their efforts to help others, that it can not only reach the White House, but also the heart of God.

I can see now that from Kansas City, to Massachusetts, and then to Florida, there He was, God in the midst of us, keeping us united through His heart to bring help to those in need. Life is not just about Patrice or my struggles, but it is about us all, and the challenges we face moment by moment. His love echoes through the years, and I for one cheer of His divine timing and brilliant light, shining on this dark illness called Fibromyalgia.

After my mother retired from the National Chronic Fatigue Association Foundation and was diagnosed with Fibromyalgia, she began a small Care, Prayer, and Share newsletter where the focus was on supporting one another in spiritual and emotional aspects of one's life. I often added poetry to the newsletters and though it was my mother's project, I was honored to have a small hand in it as well. Fibromyalgia is embedded in my family history. Beside's my mother, and myself my brother was diagnosed with both

CFS and Fibromyalgia. He has been on disability for the past twenty-five years. It has been very difficult for him to live with the emotional heartbreak of not being the primary breadwinner in the family. He was a stay at home dad and because of this, many friends and even some family members, thought he was just lazy. They had no clue about his illness and the limitations it put on him. It can be very difficult for a man to be stripped of what he thinks is part of his manliness, being the primary financial support of his family. Of course today it is not so unusual for a man to choose to be a stay at home dad, but twenty-five years ago it was not as easily accepted.

Given my family history, my experience with Fibromyalgia has been broader then most others. In fact five of my family members were attacked by this illness. One thing is for sure though, we supported and loved one another as we truly understood the day-by-day challenges. There is strength in numbers. You are NOT ALONE!

THE PRICE

What is the price, how much do I pay?
I had twenty cents but nothing today.
I'm bankrupt and hurting, my mind in a fog,
What is the price of chronic pain, fatigue and loss?

I come to the threshold of well meaning friends,
Who offer advice and pray without end.
I honor and trust them with hearts that do care,
But what is the price if the pain they can't share?

I'm humbled and broken, no strength for the day,
I offer a tear to my God by the way.
Oh, how to serve Him, to work and not tarry,
But all I can offer is my love and I'm weary.

The colors of Fibro are the blues with a cost,
The pink inflammation and the red hot spots.
There's hope in the morning until I wake with this pain,
And bend to the horror of chronic sickness again.

My hope is salvation, a new body one day.
The love of my Savior who is with me today.
And though I am broken and struggling for more,
I lay in His arms for He is my cure.

His love ever present, His heart opens wide,
For all the oppressed and all those who strive.
His grace is sufficient, the price He did pay,
His pain was endured, His cross lead the way.

No matter the price, no matter the cost,
He paid it at Calvary to save what was lost.
Through His stripes I am healed; I know what to pray,
As I wait for more healing, I will serve Him each day.

No mountain can stop me, no valley below,
Can quench my desire to serve Him and know,
The Love of the Father, the Son and the Spirit,
Is with us who suffer, and ever so near us.

CHAPTER 3

IT IS NOT JUST ACHING MUSCLES

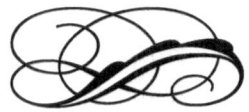

When you say aching muscles, it sounds like a nuisance and something that is manageable. Not true. While there are varying degrees of pain, many people with Fibromyalgia suffer from "pain" throughout their body, not just a dull ache. I have been one of the luckier ones. When I first got Fibromyalgia back in 1986, it started as a dull ache and did at times become intense pain. However, after seven years of suffering with it, it did become a dull ache that only flared up occasionally. It stayed that way until about five years ago. I use to wonder why people with Fibromyalgia took pain medications like Vicodin and Percocet. Now I understand. Rather than an aching body, Fibromyalgia can present with intense pain throughout the entire body, usually with the pain being more intense in certain areas. I am talking unbearable pain in your arms, legs, neck, back, and even in the face, pain so intense that only a strong pain medication can make it bearable. I often get this pain in my upper back and neck, sometimes at night in my legs. This limits my ability to walk, stand for more than an hour or so and even sit for a long period of time. There are some who have pain throughout their entire body almost on a daily basis. They could not survive without pain meds. They would go insane from the continuous pain. I know several women with Fibromyalgia who have been called drug addicts when in fact; they are taking the appropriate amount of pain medication for their level of pain. As a matter of fact, on several occasions when working as a Drug and Alcohol Clinician, I was able to advocate for several women who were actually being accused of abusing pain medication, even though it was prescribed. Evidently, some feel that if you can't see the pain, it doesn't exist. I believe that it was divine providence that these particular women were assigned to me to be evaluated, as I was ultimately able to invalidate the charges against them. One of them was actually at risk of losing custody of her child. Talk about being misunderstood and adding to their discomfort.

Now let's look at all the misconceptions about exercise and Fibromyalgia. Yes, you do need to keep moving with this illness or it does get worse, but how much is so totally misunderstood. Each person needs to figure this out for their selves by experimentation as each one of us are very different. Many doctors will simply say, "work through the pain" or do this or that exercise. This is so far from the right way to present this issue. Many try to work through the pain and end up having a severe relapse. Let me try to explain. While movement is good, it needs to be adjusted to each person's ability to move and to the severity of the Fibromyalgia. What

I have found is that when I walk or do any exercise I look at when it starts to really hurt and the fatigue level. If I try to push through the pain while greatly fatigued or when the pain greatly intensifies, I will only make myself so much worse. For me, I can usually walk about 30 minutes at my pace, which isn't really too slow. However, I can only walk up a very light incline, anything more just doesn't work for me. When I have had a busy week, or get very fatigued, sometimes I skip my walk or just walk for ten minutes. It takes a lot of trial and error to get to know your own body's signals. Every other night I work my arms with some one-pound weights and now I can do eight to ten repetitions without hurting myself. That is not to say I won't feel a little sore, but it won't push my pain level over the edge. I also do some floor exercises and know exactly how many I can do. Remember, I started all this 20 years ago. I actually started out walking 10 minutes a day and only doing 4 repetitions. It may not seem like much to a healthy person, but it keeps me going and somewhat toned. And, there are many times that I will go somewhere where I walk a lot more, like a fair or beach area. I am just careful to watch my output during the few days that follow such a day or days to be careful not to push myself into a flare up. Again, you need to be so careful with exercise and be so aware that most doctors don't have a clue. You have to find what fits you.

I will give you a good example of not paying attention to your body. I recently got the brilliant idea that I would take up Tai Chi since I had heard that it was good for Fibromyalgia. But, I did not use my own acquired understanding of how to incorporate it into my daily exercise life. So, I charged full speed ahead and did it every day for about one week, even when I felt that pain level rise and the fatigue set in. Seriously, you would think by now I would know better. Well, it brought on two months of pain and fatigue that almost just sent me over the edge. I did not think I would survive it. I would wake up every day thinking I was going to die. Obviously I did not, but it was brutal. I have yet to start taking any pain meds other than Ibuprofen, but I got close during this flare up. Each day I would think to myself, "you idiot, what were you thinking"? It has been three months since doing Tai Chi and I am just returning to what is my normal baseline.

So, when someone with Fibromyalgia says they can't do something because of their pain level, graciously accept that they can't. And if you are out somewhere and they can't continue, find them a nice spot where they can sit while you do what you have to do. I know that there are times when out with friends that I can't do all they can so I find a place where I can sit back and read and wait for them. I remember once, I rolled up in a blanket and rested on the beach while friends of mine hiked around the shore. It was a nice day for all of us. So, the person with Fibromyalgia needs to let others do what they can while they in turn find a way to take care of themselves. As for me, I don't like missing out on fun, so I always prepare for the event that I might not be able to keep up and look at alternatives to keep myself occupied and comfortable.

To sum it up, what I want people to know is that while

the pain of Fibromyalgia can be a dull ache, it more often is in the actual "pain" category. Sometimes so intense that pain meds are needed and people's lives are restricted. And, if someone doesn't walk around moaning, it doesn't necessarily mean that they are not really in pain. Keep that in mind and be careful not to judge. I have one very close friend who experiences intense pain and must take the pain medication. She only takes what she needs to take each day and nothing more then that. Only very close friends even know she has Fibromyalgia and from appearances most would never know what she struggles with each day.

Now, there are drugs known to help with Fibromyalgia pain other your typical pain meds, such as Lyrica and Cymbalta. I know people who take them and do get some relief. However, they do have a lot of side effects making them difficult for many to take. Personally, I cannot take them.

Diana Speaks:

As I was reading more of Patrice's comments on exercise, I was reminded of when I went to the pain clinic last year for the first time. The nurse began to take down my history and ask me about why I was there. As soon as I said the word "Fibromyalgia", she told me all I needed to do was exercise and that would help break down what was collecting in my body and causing pain. My heart suddenly sank as I thought, "this place will offer me no help". As time went by and the nurse continued to talk to me, the pain in my body increased and began to show on my face. I could feel the tears welling up behind my panicked eyes. I think the nurse noticed and began to realize that I was not crazy, lazy, or mentally ill. She began to get that I was suffering physically and she began to react to me in a much more compassionate way. Now I simply became Diana a new patient, not just a statistic with a little understood illness. I was the real face of Fibromyalgia sitting before her. Though I had walked in there with my makeup in place, hair done appropriately, with no visible sign of illness, she began to see past this presentation of wellness into the heart of my suffering.

The pain doctor offered no cure, but he did offer two Tramadol a day, which just takes the edge of my pain. He did, however, offer compassion and continued to ask me more about my pain. I was thankful when he talked about some treatment for my lower back. He appeared to truly want to help and continued to ask questions, digging deeper than just the Fibromyalgia. He was looking for anyway to help me with my pain. I think what made the day seem like a victory to me was the fact that I did not hold back who I was or what I was experiencing. My voice told my story and it was alive, it was acknowledged, and I saw break through on the nurse and doctor's face as they came to realize that the physical suffering of Fibromyalgia is real. Mind you, I do believe that exercise is good and can help us; it's not the first thing we want to hear, as if it's a cure all.

Fibromyalgia is not just a name; it is an illness that causes a person to wear a heavy garment of pain. It cannot remain silent and hidden or misunderstood any longer. We must become willing to be vulnerable enough to let the makeup fade and the true face of suffering be seen. Others cannot possibly understand if we are not willing to be stripped down of our emotional barriers and share our reality with them. We must tell them about this uninvited illness and hold back nothing. Our friends and family need to know more in order to understand fully and allow their compassion flow. Let your light shine but be a revealer of the darkness, while still embracing the light of God and hope in Him. Be ye not silent, but be ye known from every facet of your soul and spirit. Be true to who you are, the heights and the deepest depths of your being. Be fully engaged in life, in love, in sharing, in explaining, and in the patient revelation of truth. Only then will others begin to understand the life of one who lives with Fibromyalgia.

UN-INVITED

How loud is the pain, how much can I take?
The volume uncharted, the message to great.
How much can I handle, is the breaking point near?
How deep is the water, am I drowning in here?

Days of the gray, the black and the blue,
When pressure points throb and the mind needs renewed.
The fog is unending; the drama unfolds, a friend uninvited,
Chronic pain I know.

It's breath is too heavy; the voice is too sharp,
I'm broken and wounded from the attack in the dark.
The daylight, the noonday, the times ever changing, a friend
un-invited
Fibromyalgia engaging.

CHAPTER 4

IT IS MORE THAN JUST FATIGUE

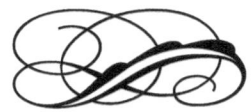

Seriously, sometimes the fatigue associated with Fibromyalgia is so bad I can't move. Fatigue with this illness comes in varying degrees at different times. But, almost always I feel some degree of fatigue. I have learned to live with it. Now, I can already hear some folks expressing how a little fatigue shouldn't keep you down, that many people have fatigue. They have no idea what they are talking about until they experience it. Yes, most of my days I can function with the mild fatigue. It is difficult, but I have found ways to do it and still enjoy life. Then there are those moderate days where I have to restrict what I do. This is when I have to make hard choices, like what I will participate in that day and what I need to eliminate. Of course, if you work like I do, work has to come first. This has greatly limited my social life. While I still care deeply for many of my friends and relatives, I simply cannot go to functions or go out with them. I just don't have the energy to do it. Having this illness often means making difficult choices.

So what does this word fatigue actually look like with Fibromyalgia? On a good day it means that I feel "sluggish", like I need a little more sleep. That is a good day. Over the years I have found ways to deal with it. I have been able to work part-time so I have to monitor my physical output around working. So far I have been successful for the most part; but it took me years to of trial and error to get to this point. On several occasions, usually out of pure frustration and desire to bring in more income, I did attempt to work a 40-hour a week job. It just never worked out. My body could pull it off for about two or three months and then it just crashed.

You are probably wondering what I mean by "crash". Well, when I attempt to push through a certain level of fatigue and pain that I know means to slow down, and I have created a schedule where there is no time in it to pull back and rest, like working full time, my body simply crashes. The fatigue especially becomes so intense and overwhelming that I can no longer function. Seriously, I can't move. There is no pushing through it, because you simply can't. When I crash and it is a really intense crash, I could be in bed and the house could be on fire and I still would not move. Nothing matters except not moving. It is such an all-consuming sense of fatigue that it feels like you have lost control of your own body. And, in a sense you have. This happens periodically even when I work part-time, but it usually only happens once every few months and only lasts for a day. But, when I attempted full time work or just keep a schedule that is too much for me, I can crash and it can last for weeks. Some people also refer to crashing as a "flare up". However, I can crash and it can be just intense fatigue but when I get a lot of pain with it, I tend to call that a flare-up. Flare-ups can be brought on by activity or sometimes they just happen.

So, what do you do when you crash or have a flare-up? Usually nothing. It doesn't make sense to fight your body at this time. It makes more sense to stay in bed, rest, and try to keep some space between yourself and stressful situations. It means time alone. It is extremely unpleasant and emotionally draining. I remember one time I was out with a friend who had known me for years. She knew I had a strong work ethic and had battled this illness for years. But still, when talking about ways I could bring more money into my home, she looked at me and told me about a woman who was undergoing chemotherapy and how she pushed through her pain and fatigue everyday to keep working. I could not believe what she had just said that to me. You see, because this illness doesn't usually affect how someone looks, they assume you are not really in any distress. How do you get across to someone that there is no pushing through when someone with Fibromyalgia crashes or has a flare-up? I guess by telling them. That is what I am attempting to do.

On the lighter side, one day I had been having what seemed like the never-ending flare-up and was desperate for relief so I went to a Catholic Healing Service. So, I finally get my time with the priest and what do you think he says. He tells me how great I look for someone who has been suffering a chronic illness for 25 years. I got back to my seat and actually started laughing. I mean what else could I do. Go beat up the priest. No, after 25 years of dealing with such comments I am getting better at handling them. Years before it was a different story. One day when I was working part-time and had gone to do an errand on a day that the pain and weakness in my legs was very bad, I used my handicapped-parking placard. As I was walking towards the store, a woman yelled at me in front of many other shoppers that I was parked in a handicapped parking space. I looked at her and told her I had a placard that she would be able to see when she got near the car. Instead she rudely shouts, again in front of other shoppers, "you are not handicapped". I was mortified. Instead of ignoring her as I probably would today, I yelled back at her out of anger. Yup, I did and immediately felt worse than if I had let it go. When I went back to work I was in tears and told my boss what had happened. She could not stop laughing and said the other woman deserved it. Still, that is not how I want to present myself to the world. But the point is that many people with Fibromyalgia suffer such comments and insults all the time. And, when you think about it, no one should question when someone has a handicap-parking placard as there are many disorders and illnesses that could cause someone to have difficulty walking long distances.

The major point that I am trying to get across is that someone with Fibromyalgia doesn't just suffer from mild fatigue; they aren't just tired. Instead it varies from day to day and when they say they don't have the energy to do something, they aren't wimping out, they really can't. And, when they say they can't work, they usually can't. It is not a choice. The fatigue can be overwhelming and all consuming and it can strongly limit someone's life. So, show some mercy.

Diana Speaks:

Speaking of fatigue, and yes it has a voice, and though it is faint and weak, it still tells a compelling story of physical and emotional struggle. Yesterday I went into my dark bedroom and stayed in a cocoon of exhaustion and pain. That was the price I paid after attending a much needed church service and lunch with my brother and sister-in-law. You might ask, "Was it worth it"? Yes, it sure was because the light of fellowship brings emotional and spiritual healing as the joy of worship and praise brings wind and air to rise upon. There has to be balance in our lives; and choices to go out and play, or in this case to pray. I may have felt weaker the day after in my body, but my inner being was blessed and refreshed. Sometimes our bodies do not react negatively to an event, we just never know. One day we do fine with an activity, and then on another day, that same event puts us in bed for a day or a week. So we gamble, making the most informed decision that we can because we need to get out of the house and create happy memories and enjoy simple pleasures, even if we have to spend the next day, or week in bed.

Take for an example my grandson. Last time I visited Kansas I decided to keep him home from day care in order to have a whole day with him. He is an active three year old and having that opportunity to be with him was worth any pain and fatigue that resulted from my physical activity that day. I chose something that was dear to me, and the joy I got from that day overrode all those sore muscles and fatigue. We learn to live with Fibromyalgia and have to find ways to make peace with our limitations. The good thing is that flare-ups pass and the sun does come out again. Resting and accepting the consequences takes practice and self-awareness. But even when I am in that cocoon of exhaustion and pain, I am never really alone. I feel the love of God's arms around me as a song begins to play in my heart; and, I glide into that melody to escape and to sleep as I wait for physical rescue. I am reminded of a song my mother wrote when I was a child. I loved rolling down the car window and partially hanging my head out so I could sing as loud as I could the words from her song.

"Peace like a river, rippling by, peace like the billowy clouds in the sky. Peace that you feel in a warm summer's breeze, in Christ you will find all of these."

Yes, I can find peace, but only when I look up and place my brokenness in the arms of a heavenly Father who I know loves me. I trust in a Savior that bore physical pain so He could truly relate to each and every one of us. For me, He is my constant companion in good times and in challenging times of fatigue and pain. I have a friend in Jesus.

CHAPTER 5

LIVING IN THE TWILIGHT ZONE

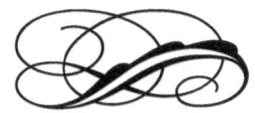

Welcome to the world of Fibro Fog. Of course you are wondering, what on earth is Fibro Fog. Well, it is an aspect of Fibromyalgia that many don't talk about and even those who suffer from it simply don't understand how and why it happens. But, it is a life stopper. It can be that one thing that can send someone with Fibromyalgia right over the edge of sanity. I know, I have been so close at times. So, what is it? It is a state of cognitive dysfunction that includes memory loss and mental confusion that can cause severe anxiety and depression. It can cause a normally self-confident, positive person to feel like a complete idiot and make them want to curl up into a ball and hide in their home. Seriously, I am not exaggerating. When this Fibro Fog is active, I can forget the names of even my own children. When working I can make mistakes that I normally would never make. Life has a surreal feel to it, like nothing is solid or real, almost like you are in a drugged state. I sometimes refer to it as living in the "twilight zone". It takes real physical and emotional effort just to get through a day feeling like this. It makes life scary and difficult to navigate. One can become paranoid and unsure of what is real and what they are imagining is real. It is devastating state to be in and most with Fibromyalgia live in this state of mind quite often. Personally, I am getting better at dealing with it but at the end of the day it often brings me to tears. Long bouts with Fibro Fog can erode me of my sense of self and the pure joy of living.

This Fibro Fog can make working very difficult. As I said, when in this state I can make mistakes that I normally would never make. The more I am familiar with a job, the easier it is to navigate the tasks when the Fibro Fog is active. For me, I try to get more rest when in this mental state. It does seem to help. And, I take a benzodiazepine, Klonopin, in very small dosages when the Fibro Fog is very active. Because it is an anti-anxiety drug, it helps slow down my thinking process so that I can think a little clearer, and keeps the anxiety at bay. This helps me cope with it without freaking out.

One of the results of Fibro Fog that many probably would not even think of is that it makes one very self aware and thus self-conscious. Normally I am a very outgoing, social person. But when the Fibro fog hits, I become very self-conscious and can overreact to stimuli in my environment. This results to my wanting to close off the world and be alone. Often this is misinterpreted as being anti-social or not caring about other's feelings. This is not true. It is simply because the Fibro Fog has taken away my coping mechanisms and created a fragile emotional state. This is especially difficult for normally strong, outgoing people to live with. For me, it has been devastating. People just don't get it. And, because I don't walk around mumbling or crying, many I know have no idea how I feel. So many people with Fibromyalgia live in this same state and suffer the same criticisms.

Consider this next time someone you know with Fibromyalgia cancels doing something. You might want to ask them if it is the pain, fatigue, or how they are emotionally feeling. If you know what it is, you might be able to help that person make some adjustments or arrangements in the activity so they can join in. Surely, if they know you understand that they are feeling emotionally fragile due to Fibro Fog and that they can trust your reaction, they may be more willing and able to engage with you. A little empathy and a soft touch go along way for someone in an emotionally fragile state.

The greatest danger of Fibro Fog is that it can cause someone who is experiencing it to develop a fear around making mistakes and experiencing that anxious feeling it can bring on. So, in order to keep some control and comfort in their lives, they will often pull back from life and seek out situations where they can be alone. This can be particularly concerning when it happens over a period of time and results in the person losing contact with those who are important in their lives. They become isolated and fearful. Often others criticize them or wonder why they no longer seek out their company. It is important when this happens to someone you love, that you reach out to the person who is suffering with Fibromyalgia and let them know you understand and encourage them to do some low key activities. Most important though, don't judge them. Just hang in there with them and they will find ways to adjust their life to living with the Fibro Fog. At least the best they can.

Speaking of not judging them, this fibro fog can sometimes cause others to misjudge what is happening to the person experiencing it. As I told you, as an Alcohol and Drug Counselor I worked with several women who were targeted as drug abusers because of their use of pain medication; when in fact, they were taking the appropriate dosages. Well, the fibro fog also played into this whole scenario. One of the complaints against one of the woman was that she sometimes appeared to be in a fog or "spaced out", sometimes not being able to recall simple information. Persons thought this woman's state of mind was caused by over dosing on her pain meds when in fact, after a long evaluation, it turned out to be Fibro Fog. Again, I believe it was divine providence that brought this woman to me to be evaluated. I was able to successfully advocate for her.

Diana Speaks:

Humor can be the saving grace while dealing with the stumbling blocks of not being able to put one thought ahead of another, let alone a foot. Being from Kansas I hold the movie "The Wizard of Oz" in very high regards. I often imagine myself as the Scarecrow simply for his known dilemma that he thought he was missing a brain. Just last week as the Fibro Fog was annoying the heck out of me; I began to sing the lyrics, "If I only had a brain". (By, Ray Bolger)

"I could while away the hours
Conferring' with the flowers,
Consulting with the rain;
And my head I'd be a scratching'
While my thoughts are busy hatching'
If I only had a brain."

I literally could not get that song out of my head and even recorded it to share with Patrice. Humor and laughter are both enormously inviting and helpful during the challenging moments with Fibromyalgia.

Does the fog lift? Yes, it can vary and there certainly are breaks or this book would not have ever been completed. But, you never know when it will subside or flare up. We can have good days too, some that feel almost normal but none for me that do not involve medication. Some days are great, although they don't come very often and are stimulated by being in the sweet spot when meds are working at their peek levels. When you are struggling, I highly recommend you seek out laughter. Such as going to a funny movie or being around witty people who you know will make you laugh. Debbie-downers can often cause you stress that can worsen or bring on a flare-up. Also, sometimes it is helpful to be around people that either have Fibromyalgia or understand your illness so you can relax. But, remember too that those who do not understand Fibromyalgia when we are dealing with a flare-up, can be as perplexed as we are. It is a confusing syndrome. I really enjoy when Patrice comes to town, as I click my heels with my "no place like home", fibro companion, because relate-ability is very important with any chronic illness. It is nice to be able to go into detail about our struggles and yet laugh at our selves too.

Now, let me share with you one very difficult day I had with Fibro Fog. Who would think a simple twenty-five minute drive to a popular little shopping area on the bay could unravel so quickly. I have to say this was one of the worst attacks on my concentration levels that I have ever experienced. Luckily I found my way there and back in one piece! So what happened you might ask? Well, I was only about ten minutes into my shopping excursion when the fibro fog, in the form of a deep mental daze, began to sweep across my mind. Let me better explain how this daze materialized this day.

I had this strange feeling of perhaps being suddenly accessorized with blinders. I could only faintly concentrate on and mentally process the twenty feet right in front of my car. It was like a dark fog was blocking out my peripheral vision. The blank stare on my face probably presented to others a look that said I should not be out of the house, let alone be driving a car. I don't remember how many times I had to say to myself, "Diana, where are you going"? I had to focus on where I was that second, where I was going, and what the next move was that I needed to make. Thank goodness it was not nighttime or forget it, with no visual cues in my surroundings, I would have turned around and just have gone back home. At one point I had to pull over and text my husband, asking him to pray for me because I was actually very frightened and concerned for myself. It was a relief to know that he would stop what he was doing and ask God to direct my path and assign angels to watch over me.

Well, I finally got to the shops on the bay and found a parking space right next to the store I had wanted to shop at, which is usually pretty hard to find. I clapped as I got out and thanked the Lord for helping me. I knew not to go to any other stores other than that one and to get right back home. I found the birthday gift for my son and was delighted with it. Before getting back into my car, I took a moment to take a picture of the boats in the marina and the palm trees that posed so delightfully against the blue fabric of the sky. We might be challenged by simple excursions, but when we make the effort, we can find true joy in the moment.

But let's just stop for a moment and look at this idea of prayer. I believe that my husband praying for me helped calm me down and be safe during this frightening mental fog experience. So I believe that there is strength in numbers, especially when we pray together. That is one of the reasons that Patrice and I decided to write this book together. We hoped to reach out to others so you would also consider the power of prayer and use it to help you live more fully with this illness and to continue to seek out healing. I have begun to pray for all of us, as a collective in this battle we call Fibromyalgia. Yes, we want a cure, but we also want a family, a gathering of women and men of all ages who also will be inspired to share in order to bring a deeper understanding to this illness. I know when I read stories from others, I suddenly get the revelation that this illness is real, and that it is not in my head. Rather, it is in my body and I am, thankfully, not going crazy.

The good news is that for me, today is a great day! I have no fog and low pain levels. So, I shout a big thank you Lord and a halleluiah for the light at the end of the fog filled tunnel for this day.

CHAPTER 6

WHY AM I SO SENSITIVE?

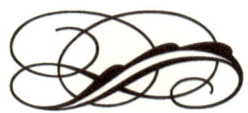

People with Fibromyalgia often experience an increased sensitivity to their environment. This can mean that sounds sound much louder than they really are, a person's allergies can intensify, and many persons actually develop new allergies and/or sensitivities to foods, drugs, and even materials used in their living space. Most people with Fibromyalgia are better off not moving to a place that is new construction as they often give off gasses that people with Fibromyalgia can't tolerate. Older places with molds and mildew can also be problematic. So they have to be extremely careful when looking for a place to live. They also need to be vigilant when trying new medications because many people with Fibromyalgia have trouble tolerating the side effects of many medications. I know that I have the strangest reactions to medications; so I am very careful when I try new ones. Often I will just start with half the recommended dosage. They are not trying to be difficult as many doctors have said to people I know. They simply cannot tolerate many of the chemicals in these drugs.

Now, when I talk about people with Fibromyalgia being sensitive to their environment, it also includes such things as large crowds; and, especially the types and volumes of noises in any given space. Too loud a noise can send someone with Fibromyalgia into a tailspin. Loud noise can hurt them, often causing a severe headache and/or confusion. They simply cannot tolerate it. They are not trying to be difficult or picky, it just is. I know for me, the confusion of a large crowd will cause my anxiety to go off the charts. I literally will flee from them. Although I really am not sure why this happens, I can only surmise that if Fibromyalgia is caused by overactive nerves in the muscles, then perhaps our entire nervous system is in overdrive. Makes sense to me and it explains the anxiety people with Fibromyalgia often experience. And I am not talking about low grade anxiety; I am talking about anxiety that feels like adrenaline is flowing throughout the body. It can be unbearable. There are medications that can help but I it is often difficult to find one that can be tolerated. Still, it is worth the effort to try.

Then there are all those general environmental issues that most people simply adjust to that those with Fibromyalgia just cannot tolerate. For example, different temperatures, inside or out, can be extremely challenging to deal with. I know in my case, I cannot tolerate the cold as it brings on muscle stiffness and soreness, which in turn triggers the fatigue. Winter can be such a challenge. I spend up to an hour a day sitting in a hot tub to relieve muscle pain and stiffness.

I lived in Florida for one year and it was the best I have ever felt. The sun on my body was so therapeutic, relieving much of the pain and stiffness. And, the water in the Gulf and in the pools was often so warm that it also was soothing to my body. I would still be there if not for a reason I cannot go into. So, each winter I am here in Massachusetts my body aches more and more. Someday I will make a warmer state my home for good.

Yet, while cold is a big issue for me, I have heard other person's with Fibromyalgia state that really hot, humid weather makes their symptoms worse. It can be different for everyone. However, I must say that most of those whom I have spoken with have stated that the cold is difficult for them. Many with Fibromyalgia do move to a warmer climate. So, even the outdoor climate can be a challenge or concern.

And then there is the food that we eat. Oh my, this can be a real issue. People with Fibromyalgia are known to suffer with so many different food sensitivities and/or stomach ailments such as Irritable Bowel Syndrome, GERD, and acid reflux. Why? I have never really heard this connection addressed, but it sure is common. I would imagine that it has to do with food sensitivities and allergies. I wonder also if given our esophagus is a muscle and other muscles are used to swallow and digest our food, if these muscles are affected by the Fibromyalgia making swallowing and digesting food difficult. But whatever the connection is, many with Fibromyalgia do suffer from some sort of digestive issues.

Now, try to imagine just for a moment how the challenge of trying to cope with all these sensitivities can affect your physical and emotional state. Physically you can become stressed and fatigued, feeling worn out and irritable. Emotionally you can feel vulnerable, anxious, and at times unable to cope, sometimes resulting in a breakdown in one's ability to communicate with others. When the struggle has gone on for a long period of time, one can lose a sense of who they are and what their strengths are. They begin to doubt their ability to move forward and can get stuck in these negative emotions. Often in search of a quiet place that does not feed into their anxiety, people with Fibromyalgia will isolate even more. They will find a safe, quiet, and controlled place and just park themselves there. I know I do it often. The result is more isolation from friends and family that can lead to feelings of aloneness and helplessness. Add this to the pain, fatigue, Fibro Fog, and many other symptoms people with Fibromyalgia must cope with and it can take such an emotional toll on a person.

Diana Speaks:

When a simple lunch with a friend suddenly turns into a game of over-active adrenaline pinball, it can be very discouraging not only for the person across the table watching this take place, but also for me, myself and I. I try so hard to hide what is going on, and often I can, but at other times I simply fail at this hide and seek game of illusion. Being apologetic often gives way to internal anger, as the fight for simple pleasures can be stolen from me at times. So, why was

I having this struggle? Why did I feel like getting up and running out to my car? Fibromyalgia, that is why. The noises around me seemed so loud and over whelming that it became difficult to even compose a logical sentence. I keep telling myself to relax, take a breath, but when the adrenaline surges and the current takes over, it's a raging engine that will not stop or become silent, no matter how many times I try to talk myself down from the emotional cliff. Frustration sets in and even trying to explain what's happening is exhausting.

So, you might wonder, how I convinced myself to go out and join the world knowing this might happen? Well, step one was the invitation that came from my friend. It often takes coaxing to get me out of the house. I had to choose to leave the comfort of my room where my environment is totally in my control because I needed adventure. I have dark curtains on the windows and the steady hum of a fan to drown out any fluctuations of sounds and a filter for too much light. I never know when I go out with a friend how I will feel, but it's worth it to have companionship once in a while. Even though it was a struggle and I had a tailspin in a restaurant at the mall, I had fun. I shared with you the complications that can arise just from lights, sounds and environmental changes as an example of what people with Fibro might encounter.

Sometimes people can get offended when they do not understand how simple changes in sound, light, and temperature can affect us so intensely. It might seem as if we can just choose not to react this way. I feel as if I am walking on eggshells with a backpack of guilt attached to me while I am in this over load state of emotion. This is one of the reasons Patrice and I wanted to write this book, so family, friends, husband, and wives of those with Fibromyalgia could learn more about how this illness affects their loved ones. We wanted to validate that all these sensitivities are not all in their loved one's heads. Reading similar stories from others gives validity to each relationship and circumstance from other perspectives.

So you can imagine by what I have said that socializing is one of the most difficult things for me to do. Others may not have the same issues as I do, as symptoms from one person to another can vary. That's where this illness can be so cruel because just going to church is even quite the challenge. Not always, but sometimes, it feels as if I have had my fingers in an electrical socket the whole time I am out and about with people. Then when the event ends, I suddenly feel set free but exhausted from the over active sensitivities I just encountered. There often is a price to be paid associated with any invitation to do something with others. I avoid it most of the time and I am sure I must appear as if I do not care, but I do. I just have this ailment, Fibromyalgia, which has attached itself to me and often will not let me enjoy the company of others. Now I have given you an example of one challenging time that ended up well pleasing once that panic attack ended. In this book we share our worst times, but too we have many fun and joyful moments so as these examples may seem harsh they can vary. Finding balance with Fibro and with life is so important. Getting out of the house even with challenges is still great medicine.

When I am going through one of those deeply intense times when all my sensitivities are on high alert, I try to take the focus off of myself and rather focus on God and His mercy. I often say to myself, "God is good and I am loved". This takes the focus off of me long enough for Him to begin to bring peace to my situation. It helps me to go to a private place and put on soft music. For me, it is Christian music that calms my nerves and brings something wonderful. Sometimes all I can say is "Help me Jesus". He always does, and the love flows over me like a warm summer breeze. Gods Word too is a dear companion. I do struggle with feelings of guilt because I tend to isolate more then what is good for me. Now...

Tic Tock, it's time to drop the guilt and all the clatter.
It is what it is, I am what I am, a survivor in times that matter.
I may not be the life of the party, or even show up at all,
But in my prayer corner I'm often a warrior
Facing giants in times of battle.

CHAPTER 7

I LOOK JUST AWFUL

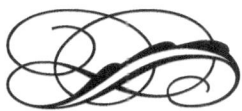

While Fibromyalgia may be an invisible illness, it can still have an effect on the way a person looks. What I mean by that is that it can cause some subtle changes in a person's appearance that can strongly affect how they feel about themselves. For example, when someone has been struggling day after day with fatigue and pain, it can present as someone being very tired. They can look drawn, pale, but not really sick. It is almost like they have lost their "glow" or that sparkle in their eye. Very often friends or family will make comments like "you look tired" or "you look sad or unhappy". Well, yes we are tired and a bit unhappy, but because we are fighting an ongoing battle with a chronic illness.

Two of the most common complaints I have heard about physical changes that people with Fibromyalgia struggle with are weight gain and dark bags and circles under their eyes. I know too some of it may sound frivolous and petty to be concerned about these two physical changes, but to the person dealing with them, it is not. How would you like to be in great physical shape and suddenly gain 20, 30, 40 pounds or more and find it almost impossible to lose it. Believe me, you would not like it. It feels bad. So why does it happen? Well, who really knows for sure; but I would bet that not being able to move as you once could has a lot to do with it. People with Fibromyalgia simply cannot exercise like they once were able to. As I mentioned, I was an aerobics instructor in the best shape I had ever been when I got sick. I once weighed 120 pounds, perfect for my 5' 4" frame. Now I struggle with 145 to 152 pounds. I hate it. It doesn't feel good carrying around this extra weight. And even though I still manage to walk on the treadmill for 30 minutes a day, although not at a very quick pace, or walk for 30 minutes or more, I struggle to lose it. And I know that there are many people with Fibromyalgia that are a lot worse off than I am and cannot walk at all. To make matters worse, most of us are not eating much more than we use to. It's very difficult to feel this helpless about your own body.

Now, I will admit this, people who feel fatigued by a chronic illness will often crave sugar. I use to notice at some of the support groups that I attended that almost everyone came with a sweet; then, I realized, I also did. It finally dawned on me that these sugary treats served two purposes. First, the sugar gave us energy. Second, I know that I got some emotional enjoyment from the sweets. Now I know these are two very bad reasons for eating it; but, when you feel down and fatigued for a long period of time your emotional defenses become very weak. And when this illness keeps you isolated and unable to do anything you use to enjoy, eating a chocolate cake with vanilla ice cream can give one a temporary, albeit not so healthy, emotional lift. So, yes, this tendency to eat sweets may play a very small part in gaining weight. However, even when I do watch what I eat, the weight is extremely difficult, and seems at times impossible, to lose. Presently, I am slowly working on losing some weight by being aware of what and how much I eat, by moving as much as I can, and by paying careful attention to my emotions. But for most of us with Fibromyalgia, it is an ongoing battle.

Oh yes, then there are those unsightly dark circles and bags under the eyes. I have to admit, these bother me the most. If I had the money for plastic surgery, I would have them removed. They make me look older and tired. And really, many people get these as we age and even movie stars have them. So, it is just my thing. I really hate them and have heard others with Fibromyalgia talk about how they struggle with dealing with the dark circles and bags under their eyes. And, honestly, I have not found anything that makes them better. I do use make-up to cover them up, but they still show. Over the years I have heard of different products that do help, but they are way too expensive for someone on a fixed income. Again, there is this sense of helplessness. So what does a girl (or guy) do? They work on accepting them. It is all you can do. It doesn't mean I have to like it though, but you can come to terms with it.

One of the other physical changes that I have difficulty

dealing with is how this disease affects my hair. All right, I know some are saying "big deal", but wait a minute; it is still a loss, and one you have to look at in the mirror all the time. I use to have long, healthy brown hair. Now it is often dry, brittle, and unmanageable. In all honesty, this really makes me self-conscious. I do use a good shampoo and hair color to make it look the best I can, but forever is gone the beautiful hair I once had. Some others with Fibromyalgia have told me they simply cut their hair short because it is so unmanageable.

On the surface all these changes might seem petty to some, but to the person whose body is changing, it is not trivial. How we look can affect our self-esteem. It is just natural. I know in my heart that I am the same person and that many have it so much worse than I do, but the loss of my physical appearance is real to me and so many others that struggle with this illness. All I can say is that, again, it is a matter of accepting the losses and somehow finding peace with it. For me, I try to focus more on my relationship with the people around me and with God. My real value lies with who I am inside, not what my body looks like at any given moment. But, I will admit, it is an ongoing battle that I only recently have gotten some real peace around. And that peace comes from deepening my relationship with a God that loves me, no matter what.

So, how can you help that person struggling with their physical appearance? Just love them. That is all you can do. Never criticize them on these issues. Actually, we should never criticize anyone on these types of issues, ever. If they talk about any of these issues to you and you have some ideas, share them; but, only if they are looking for help and only in a kind and empathic way.

Diana Speaks:

Mirror, Mirror on the wall....Stop! Yes there are times I just have to move on and come to peace over some changes in my appearance and not give it so much attention. Weight gain is more common because of lack of movement when the pain is driving the car. That is when I want to say, "Jesus, take the wheel". There is a kind of surrender that takes place that is actually very healthy for me. I hear Him encourage me and re-direct me to wiser choices. I admit I do feel better when eating right and exercising so I keep trying to follow His lead while getting my mind off the mirror. I notice it's just a distraction and as I age I want to be thinking about others and loving well like Jesus does.

It is good that I can put the mirror of who I once was down and simple move into the present time where the focus can peacefully change to others. To stare in a mirror and relent about what I use to look like, excludes the group of people I can still be a blessing to. I can do for others with much more ease things that I often find difficult to do for myself. There is energy in blessing others as an extension of God's love that is vastly more powerful and enjoyable then mourning for exterior changes. I had seen this illness take its toll on my mother as she went from a beautiful model to beautiful mentor who lost her looks but gained admiration from the thousands of people she helped during even her greatest times of pain and fatigue. She may have gained a lot of weight, but all who knew her saw a heart that was golden with the promise of a life ever after with no more pain or illness to her name. There she resides now with her new body and her mansion in the heavenly sky. So...

Mirror, mirror, you are not on my wall,
The face of the saints is my visual call.
No more of the me, the my, and the mirror,
It's onto the group to give love from the Savior.
His face is refreshing, His promise is true,
A new body awaiting, and one that's renewed.
The earth is His footstool as I rest in His fullness,
No longer am I, but a WE to influence.

CHAPTER 8

SAYING GOODBYE

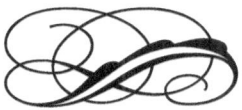

So now, hopefully, you better understand some the physical challenges of Fibromyalgia and get a sense of the emotional impact they can have on the person with this illness. Ah, but it doesn't end there. It is just the beginning. There are so many changes and losses that a person with Fibromyalgia must cope with. Life for them will never be the same. Letting go and saying goodbye will become the norm for them at many different levels at different periods of their lives. There are so many losses, so much pain and disappointment.

To start, this culture puts a high value on how a person makes a living, what kind of work they do. This is often taken away from a person with Fibromyalgia. Personally, I went from working three jobs, all which I really enjoyed, to being housebound, unable to provide for my family. Before I got sick, I had such hope for the future. I had this strong sense that I could succeed at almost anything I seriously took on and that I would become financially independent. You can't imagine how it feels to have two young children and not have the energy to get out of bed and work in order to provide for them. But, it just wasn't about provision; it was about being a useful, creative, human being who was able to pay their own way. I loved working. I loved getting a paycheck and paying my own way. Well, that was gone. It was humiliating, anxiety provoking, and confusing. Who was I that I should be in this position. Imagine the pain of not being able to give your children even the bare necessities of life. Try to imagine the fear and anxiety you would feel when you did not have enough food or didn't know where you would live. It was a living nightmare. So bad, in fact, that for about a six month period I awoke every night at about 2 or 3 a.m. in sheer panic, feeling like I could not breathe. At the time I did not understand what was happening. But now I look back and understand. I was sick, alone, broke, and scared. And, all my fear was manifesting when I went to sleep, when I let down my guard. Again, prayer was my anchor. I would grab my bible and read Psalm 91 until the fear subsided and I could go back to sleep. Psalm 91 is a prayer of God's protection. It helped me through the toughest times. So, I had to say goodbye to my work, to that part of me that expressed itself through my work. I had to say goodbye to my ability to provide for my children and myself. I had to say goodbye to that American Dream of working hard and having a good life.

Now for those of you that think that people on disability love to sit around doing nothing and collect their checks. Think again. Certainly there are those who abuse the system, but really, do you think most people enjoy trying to live on $800 to $1400 a month? We are constantly broke. Get it, we have no money, we are poor. Seriously, how can people think that anyone would want that? And, do you really think that anyone would want to depend on food stamps to eat. Think again. It is embarrassing for most people. These programs are a life saver but most people on them would love to be off them. It just takes something away from your soul when you have to rely on the government to survive. But what is the alternative? So try to be sensitive and understand that many on disability yearn to be working and experience the satisfaction of receiving a paycheck and using their talents and abilities to support themselves. Again, there is often a negative emotional impact on the person with Fibromyalgia when they cannot support themselves and have to say goodbye to their careers and perception of what being a success is all about. Show some mercy and if you are blessed financially, think about blessing someone with a chronic illness and limited resources. It would be very much appreciated.

There are other loses that someone with Fibromyalgia must face. Often it is the ability to mother or father their children. Often given their limited energy and ability to move about, activities with their children are limited. Also, people with a chronic illness almost always do not have the finances to do the simple things with their children, like go to the beach or see a movie. There just isn't any money. Again, this can be emotionally challenging and adds to the list of things that can eat away at one's self esteem.

Then there are those personal individual losses. For me it was my love of movement like walking outside, riding a bike, and most of all, dancing. I use to take these activities for granted. I don't anymore. When taken away, I had such a hole in my being. I loved to walk outdoors, rain or shine. It made me feel alive. I often prayed while walking, being close to nature made me feel close to God. Ah, but dancing was my real love. I use to dance to anything, play music and I would dance. When life got rough, I would get lost in dancing. It was good for me both on an emotional level and physically. When I got really sick, I could not dance and I could not walk, let alone ride a bike. There went my emotional outlets, my way of coping with life. I did not think I would survive.

So what do you do when what you love about yourself or life ceases to be, you say goodbye and work through the darkness that follows. Darkness, oh yes, there is almost always darkness, emotional distress. For me, again, it was through prayer. I relied on my own relationship with God and the prayers of others as I trudged through all these changes. Eventually I found some ways to cope. For example, I put a lounge chair outside under a tree, surrounded by wild flowers, in my back yard and spent much of my day out there surrounded by living, beautiful creations rather than in front of a television. At night I would lie there and look at the stars. I remember one summer the sun set right behind my back yard and the entire backyard would turn a brilliant pink as the sun set almost every night for an entire summer. People would come over just to view it or stand in the middle of it. It was incredibly beautiful. I would just lie on that lounge chair and bask in that pink hue. Guess what, I actually got better that summer. Being outside, surrounded in prayer, and working through my losses to acceptance helped my health to improve. Sometimes I would even play some music and dance just a little bit. For people with Fibromyalgia, this dance with loss and acceptance can be ongoing as their conditions changes with flare-ups and periods of relief. It is a dance that can confuse others because it does change and is not predictable. So know, if you care for someone with this illness, periods of seemingly good health with sudden changes to physical challenges are the norm. And this can affect the person emotionally, so mood changes can also be the norm. Just allow for this unpredictability and don't let it freak you out. Just be flexible and proactive in helping this person engage in life at their pace.

Diana Speaks:

You had me at "Hello", is a line from a movie I saw years ago that was spoken by a women who fell in love at first sight. As Patrice introduced to us the salutation of saying good-bye to so many things we held and cherished so dearly, I could not help but think of this line. She said hello to love, and now we must say good-bye to only some of the things we once did, as we say "Hello" to something new.

Let me expound now on what comes next. I contemplated on the analogy of turning a new page, or going into a new chapter of my life. I want to embrace the changes and the challenges of the courageous move I can take by turning the page and starting a new chapter in my life. It is in my perspective that life can take on new meaning as I start to write upon this chapter as I expound upon my own personal life story. You have heard that old saying about turning lemons into lemonade. Well, we can do the same thing with our lives. They might look different, but they can still be good. We can offer our experiences to others in the desire to share the whole truth, nothing but the truth, so that we might explore the new doors that one who lives with Fibromyalgia is able to walk through. By writing this book, I am walking through one of those new doors. But let me reflect for just a moment on what once was so very dear to me in my life.

Several years ago I was a wedding photographer and loved my career very much. Though I had been struggling with Fibromyalgia for decades, I found something that only took one day a week outside my home to do and manage. Editing on the other hand took two more weeks at my computer. Even though I could manage this career, I remember having panic attacks often as I anticipated the physical strain of actually photographing my next wedding assignment. When I had to finally give this up because of the pain and fatigue, I thought I lost what I was passionate about and my creative outlet. This made me feel as if I was not being productive. It was a hard pill to swallow. People often ask me to return to photography; but as of yet, I still have not felt strong enough, nor God's lead in that direction. Yes I thought it was a loss, but now this moment I see it was a storybook adventure that I was so very happy to experience. It makes me happy to see all the locations my team and I got the privilege to go. Yes, I did have a team that worked with me. I am so grateful to them for helping me realize my dream. It was a goodbye but not the end of my creative story.

Healing from these good-byes can be difficult if we are only looking backwards. Embracing a new life is filled with uncertainty but even with an illness it does not mean we cannot have marvelous new adventures. Patrice described so beautifully the scene in her back yard as she exchanged the gloom of the inward isolation with the beauty of creation. She talked about how she found more of the meaning of life by reaching beyond her physical confinement. Then God did His part, didn't He? He painted the sunset and His palate glowed with the golden, warm pink tones that enveloped her back yard. Her choice to say goodbye to sitting in the darkness of her house opened up a glorious expanding image of what is truly to come. You might say she got a glimpse of heaven. She even testified to the fact that she physically felt better as she stepped into this anointed atmosphere. Oh for God's healing touch and His presence.

We get to experience God in so many ways that we can take it for granted. Then when life gets difficult and stays that way for a long time, we can become accustomed to the dark side of gloom and miss the accompanying melody of the Harvest moon so large and beautiful that it can take our breath away. In other words, we can get stuck. By going outside Patrice became unstuck. I can truthfully say that I can begin to see myself sitting beside Patrice, there in her backyard, her haven of rest and restoration, sipping a glass of lemonade as we listen to Christian music. I can imagine that our conversations would be centered around the naturally, yet spiritually inspired moments of grace. That is I, making a choice to say hello, right after the goodbyes. I am trusting God to put His hand on mine as I turn the pages of what was and embark upon the adventure of what will be as long as I have God leading me onward. Lord, you had me at Hello, and I thank you for the hope of new horizons and sunsets to come.

CHAPTER 9

I CAN'T TAKE IT ANY LONGER

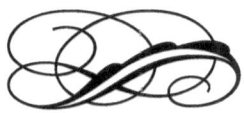

Now let's look at what many people with Fibromyalgia often struggle with but sometimes do not tell anyone about, depression. It is referred to as secondary depression because it is the result of the illness and all the changes this illness brings into a person's life. And it is a depression that can go very deep. I am not talking about a simple case of the blues, but rather a state of intense despair. The problem is that in this society depression is somewhat stigmatized so it is difficult to talk about. But the struggle is real and sometimes dangerous. Some of you are wondering why I say dangerous. Well, on many occasions when talking to someone who is going through a difficult flare-up of Fibromyalgia, I hear the words "I can't take this any longer". Most of the time it is just an expression used to convey how bad the person feels. However, sometimes it means that a person is considering "suicide". There I said it. When Fibromyalgia is severe over a long period of time, suicide is sometimes considered as an option for relief. And I will put myself out there and tell you that I thought of it often. Seriously, it sometimes feels like the right thing to do. Right now there are those that are thinking it is just a cop out. But wait; let's take a closer look at the multiple issues this illness brings into a person's life that maybe you never considered.

To start, you have all the physical suffering: unrelenting pain and fatigue, Fibro Fog, and all kinds of sensitivities. There is also a long list of other physical symptoms that many suffer from. Some of them are headaches, stomach problems like irritable bowel syndrome, acid reflux and Gerd, difficulty breathing when the chest muscles are fatigued, loss of balance, tingling in the limbs and the list just goes on and on. Add to all these physical challenges the emotional challenges and losses, economical, social, and personal, that someone with Fibromyalgia must live with and you have a life disrupted, filled with uncertainty and struggles. Can you imagine living with all this over a long period of time? Are you getting the picture? And, add to all this that many think that others would be better off without them. After all, what good are you if you are stuck in bed? It can be devastating. I consider myself a very strong person and I have a deep and steady faith in Jesus, but I still struggle with thoughts of suicide, not often, but on occasion. I use to feel guilty but I don't anymore. I have come to understand that depression often goes hand and hand with this illness and I know that I do my best to keep it under control. But after a long, relentless flare up, I just feel I can't stand it for another moment. The really sad reality is that even as a Christian, I often have no one to say this to. Being able to admit that you are struggling with depression and/or feeling suicidal helps tremendously. But even many mature Christians hold the view that if you are right with God you would not get depressed. I guess they haven't read the Psalms where different bible characters express their emotional despair. And, a body in constant pain can deplete the feel good chemicals in the brain, like Dopamine and Serotonin. It is no wonder that the result can be a very deep, ongoing depression.

Well, how one handles depression is a very private matter. I know that for me just accepting it makes it easier to cope with. I admit I am depressed and express my pain to a few people I know can handle it. People like my therapist and my friend Diana in Florida. She also suffers from Fibromyalgia and I can tell her my very deep thoughts without her judging me or freaking out. So yes, you really need to be careful when you are deep in depression who you talk to. Many people can't handle such a conversation, so don't go there. Knowing who can and who can't listen to your thoughts is important. And remember, it doesn't make someone "bad" just because others can't "deal "with where you are at. It is ok.

Of course, there is always medication for an ongoing depressive episode and rather than suffering and putting yourself in emotional turmoil, it might be a good option to consider. As for me, I do take a small amount of an anti-depressant and it does help, except when the flare- up goes into months long. Then I have to take out all my coping mechanisms and put them in place. For me, I first talk to my friend Diana and my therapist about it. I also find going to the movies enjoyable and easy on the body, so I seek out some fun movies to attend. A good book in a quiet environment also helps relieve the distress. But, I must say, my faith and prayer has kept me going when I just felt I could not go on. I even enlist the prayers of others for added support. I can't stress too much how having a personal relationship with Jesus has saved my life. There have been times when I was ready to just give up when I could actually feel His presence and was then able to move forward. Or, there have been times when I would express my pain to God and just the right person would call or drop over. This is not an illness I can fight alone.

I can remember recently having one of the worst flare-ups I have ever had. It went on for months and the symptoms were worse than I can ever remember them being. So, I actually made a decision to take my own life one year from then when my life insurance would allow suicide as a means of death. So, here I am sitting in church, singing to God, and I have decided that I could not live with this illness anymore. You see I believe that God would have received my soul even if I took my own life because he loves me and knows my heart. Anyway, during the service you could actually feel the Holy Spirit flowing through the room. It was a warm gentle sense of His presence and all I could do was cry. Then this gentleman across from me spoke out loud a message from God. Now when he did, you could feel a change in the atmosphere, Jesus was now present. I mean He always is, but this was in a more tangible way. Well, as soon as that gentleman spoke the word that God had given him, I stopped crying and all thoughts of suicide left. God had honored my presence and my turning to Him by increasing the Holy Spirit's presence to break off the thoughts of suicide. I always tell people, do not run from God when life gets tough even if you think He doesn't really like what you are thinking or doing, run to Him. There you will find peace. Truly this works. When you run to God, He draws closer to you. The bible states that when we are weak He is strong. How very true this is. But the bottom line is, that when living with a chronic illness like Fibromyalgia, or with any other chronic illness, you often have to dig deep inside of yourself and find that spiritual part of you that can help you cope, to help you live your life with some degree of hope and peace.

Diana Speaks:

Everything and everyone ever born has a story to tell. We all want someone to take the time to hear ours. We are human beings who have an illness; but we have to work at not letting it define who we actually are. I call this my authentic nature, or self. Before Fibromyalgia, I was just Diana and all those fibers of memories live, linger, and paint a unique picture from the canvas of my whole life, not just the life inside of any particular ailment. I am not Fibromyalgia. And, though at times it seems to imprison me, it still should not define me. I have to take pleasure in small victories and allow myself to find joy in simple things. When you really think about it, we all should live like this. I also have to take medication for depression because without it, even a small challenge seems overwhelming. If medication can help you, then investigate that avenue with your doctor. Yes, there are other ways to combat depression, such as prayer, meditation, nutrition, physical exercise, fellowship and new things to look forward too. I find that by taking a little from this and a little from that, I am creating a kind of teamwork approach that helps me function much better. Some days I almost feel "normal", though many days I find I am still taking baby steps, while other days I seem to move through the day with much more ease.

Even with Fibromyalgia, not every day is filled with obstacles. There are days when I feel good, almost normal, and wonder what I can do to stay this way. Because I tend to feel more stress and have more days that are challenging, when I have a good day I will often over analyze it and wonder if something is wrong with me because I feel good. Can you see the flaw in this thinking? I can because I am moving into guilt or a stress thought process by bringing up a negative-positive statement. Then I miss the good day. I have to remind myself that there is nothing wrong with me when I feel good. I need to just enjoy the day. Our thoughts can bring on undue stress that can lead to depression.

I have discovered that sometimes the mental choices I make can help or hurt also. As I began this section I stated that everything has a story. Even my pillowcase has a story. I look at the fabric and wonder where did it originate? Is it cotton? If so, it began with a seed put into the ground, then the rain watered it, then the sun brought it forth from the ground and it sprung up reaching to the sky in adoration. From there it is passed through human hands who each had a story themselves. On to manufacturing, dying of the material, and then the pattern is created. A friend made my particular pillowcase and I can just imagine her now as she cut out the material and sat at her sewing machine to make my pillowcase. Goodness, even the thread has a story, doesn't it?

What I am trying to bring to light is that there are so many wonderful things we can pass the time thinking about and exploring even from our easy chair. If I focus on the darkness then I end up in a box suffocating. I have to learn to be proactive in what I choose to think about. I often find myself dwelling on my illness or pain. When I do this I have to stop and ask God to cover my thoughts with His and draw me into prayer for others so my focus is not always on myself. I can imagine that my prayers can reach a loved one a thousand miles away and thus create a wonderful ripple effect in their lives that just might make a difference. What I have found to be the most helpful is when I begin my day with worship music. While waiting for my pain medication to kick in, I sing to the Lord and the atmosphere changes. Rejoicing for me has become a sweet place that offers healing from the Lords presence. There are so many anointed threads that make up the fabric of my life but the best of them all is the garment of praise.

To appoint unto them that mourn in Zion, to give unto them beauty for ashes, the oil of joy for mourning, the garment of praise for the spirit of heaviness; that they might be called trees of righteousness, the planting of the Lord, that he might be glorified. Isaiah 61:3 KJV

CHAPTER 10

THESE MOOD SWINGS ARE BRUTAL

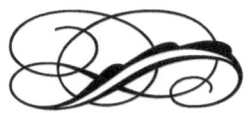

One of my greatest challenges with this illness is the mood swings and how they affect my social interactions. There are days that I feel like hiding in my house just so I don't have to interact with anyone. Why, you are probably wondering? Because when I am not feeling well and/or in pain, I can become a very "nasty" version of myself.

I have always valued kindness, patience, and empathy in how I personally interact with others, whether socially or at work. Well, after days of intense pain, fatigue and dealing with Fibro Fog, I can actually become very short tempered and even nasty at times when interacting with others. This is one of my greatest challenges; how to cope with what I am feeling and not lash out at others. I have improved greatly over the years, but it will continue to be a challenge for me. Here are a few of the things I have done to try to help me cope with this challenge.

First, acknowledge that you are feeling that edginess and be on full alert for situations that could set you off. This has helped to stop and think about my responses before they came out the wrong way. Second, when I feel really edgy, or just plain down, I will take a small amount of anti anxiety medication to help me relax so that I can cope better. Also, I let people who know me know that I am feeling edgy and anxious and ask them ahead of time to forgive any sharpness in my tone that they may detect. Finally, I just do my best to be aware of my tone of voice and acknowledge when I may be in danger of "losing it" and try to walk away from the situation until I can better handle it. As I said, it is an ongoing challenge but I have come a long way in dealing with it. The awareness of how I can present when I feel edgy and down has helped me enormously in regards to controlling myself. But let me tell, it is tough.

So try to understand and remember, someone who is dealing with ongoing pain, fatigue, or other aspects of an illness, will be prone to mood swings and may come across at times as short tempered, sarcastic, or just plain impatient. Try to have some empathy and patience with them. If you need to correct them, do so in a kindly manner. And, if they apologize for something they said, a tone of voice, or a way they acted that you now understand is caused by coping with the illness, be quick to forgive and don't take it personally. The human body can only take so much and know that someone who has a "chronic illness" uses an enormous amount of energy just attempting to cope with it. The result can be a tired, cranky, and short-tempered human being.

Diana Speaks:

Most of the time, I live in a happy-go-lucky bubble. It feels as if it's a protective covering that God placed around me for as long as I can even remember. My grandmother Bertie told me that I was always smiling, even as a baby. But she elaborated about a time as a toddler that I was very sick, and was given a medicine that I had an allergic reaction to as well. Grandma said that I totally lost my smile during that time. She knew to pray for me and soon my sickness was gone and my smile returned.

What I would like to express here is that love, and prayer certainly help tremendously during a bad flare with any illness. Compassion can bring a smile back to a loved one who is suffering. Even now with my husband, when I am in a bad way, he can see it in my eyes and in the missing smile. When this happens his whole demeanor becomes that of protector and guardian. I can feel so horrible but when he turns up the volume of love, it brings a smile to my face no matter how I feel his love can heal. There is such a powerful energy all around us that we can tap into that can change the atmosphere.

Then there are times I want people to read my mind, and just know that I feel bad. But that is not doing them justice. Let others know when you are low so they get the opportunity to extend the hand that heals.

CHAPTER 11

HELP, I AM BEING MISUNDERSTOOD AND "ARRESTED"

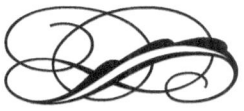

I just have to tell you this story. It really shows how someone with Fibromyalgia, and other similar illness, can be totally misunderstood. So, here goes.

Just a few months ago a friend of mine got arrested for "Driving Under the Influence". I truly believe she wasn't under the influence of anything. The day it happened she had just picked up a new car and was having some trouble adjusting to the new brakes; so, she admits that she may have swerved a few times when she was slowing down. Then at one point she nicked the bumper of someone's car. There was no damage as she was driving very slowly. She said she was preoccupied with getting use to the new brakes that she misjudged the distance between her and the car in front of her. Now, keep in mind she was only driving about 20 miles per hour the entire time. Well, apparently the person driving behind her told the police that she was swerving when she was driving, a fact that she readily admitted to, explaining that it was a result of getting use to the new brakes that somehow did not feel quite right. Now here is where things could have gone so differently if she did not have Fibromyalgia.

She was then asked to take a physical sobriety test. Now she knew she could not pass it. Like many people with Fibromyalgia, she had an unsteady gait and weakness in her legs that would absolutely prevent her from standing on one foot for any amount of time or even walking toe to toe. Therefore, she failed the test. Now I still think given that the police saw her handicap plate, they would have realized she might be telling the truth and tried another test. They did not and when she told them she had Fibromyalgia, they immediately asked what meds she took. Being an honest person, she told them she took pain meds but explained that she took her last dose at 6 a.m., 5 hours earlier. The police then began to search her car. I think they automatically assumed she was abusing drugs. Well, they did find her pains meds in her purse but she also had her prescription with her, so she did not get cited for having them on her. This is where I truly believe the police could have done better.

At this point they handcuffed her and arrested her. All the while, she is offering to take a drug test to prove there wasn't enough pain medicine in her system to inhibit her ability to drive. She did take a Breathalyzer and passed. She explained that she and her doctor had developed a system of taking her pain meds so it would never put her in danger. I know for a fact that she would never drive under the influence. For me, it is the way they treated her that really bothers me, not the fact that they arrested her. After all, they could see that she was handicapped and she was being honest and cooperative while asking that they please drug test her. But instead they treated her like a common criminal and never attempted to understand the reality of her not being able to pass the sobriety tests that they asked her to do. This really bothers me as I could not pass them either. I think the police need to find ways to drug test persons they suspect of using so that innocent people don't have to go through the arrest procedure.

Another issue I think that may have caused the police to move forward with the arrest is that they saw that this woman had a lot of anxiety and movement, perhaps misinterpreting it as drug use. It is not uncommon for persons with Fibromyalgia to become agitated and anxious when under stress. After all their bodies are already stressed from the pain and fatigue, so it is no wonder that an added stress like being arrested, can just turn up that anxiety to a much higher level. In addition, when your arms are hurting and they are yanked behind your back, the pain can be intense. Then there are those wonderful wooden benches and beds with no mattress that can also ratchet up the pain level, sometimes to unbearable intensities. I know that this woman was in such intense pain that she tried to fall asleep while lying on this brick hard bed. She had reached her coping level. Again, the police thought she was falling asleep from drug use. They simply would not address her disability. So what could have happened here that could have made things easier for this woman? First the police should have taken the time to listen, no matter how anxious she presented as. I believe they should have done a drug test, as it would probably have cleared her. Better communication may have kept it out of court. Recently the case went to court and the DUI was dropped.

I told you this story just to drive home how misinterpreted the symptoms of this illness could be. Of course this is extreme, but experiences similar to this do happen. I think if people like the police better understood Fibromyalgia and perhaps other disabling illnesses, they would be able to better handle the situations. Remember I told you about the several women I was able to advocate for; well, if I had not understood this illness, I would not have been able to do so and one of them may have lost custody of her child. It is important to help people understand Fibromyalgia. Lack of knowledge can result in devastating outcomes as a result of misinterpreted situations.

Diana Speaks:

As Patrice shares this woman's plight of being arrested and charged with Driving Under the Influence due to such misinterpretation of her behavior, I feel compelled to share with you how we can also misinterpret what our own bodies are doing. This happens when we attribute everything going on in our bodies to the Fibromyalgia, when in fact, it could be something else altogether.

Recently, the Fibromyalgia was screaming so loudly and blowing up such a smoke screen that I was not aware of another condition going on in my body for about 8 months. I have since learned that not everything is Fibromyalgia. But, that this illness does sometimes blind our perception when other things in our bodies begin to change. Let me explain.

Alarm bells were ringing concerning my mid-section enlarging and getting hard. I associated it with digestive issues common to Fibromyalgia. I experimented with removing gluten and dairy from my diet, which did help with the bloating, so I thought that was all I needed to do. A few weeks ago I decided to go to a doctor who specializes in the digestive tract and they ordered a cat scan to see if something else was going on. Two days before I was scheduled to go on a cruise, I was called into the doctor's office "immediately". Let me tell you, when you get a phone call from a doctor who wants to see you the next day, you know there is a major issue involved. My brain fog from the Fibromyalgia suddenly was gone at the realization that I possibly had a life threatening condition going on that was not related to Fibromyalgia.

I was going to go alone to the doctor, but fear began to set in, not only in myself but my husband Danny as well. He accompanied me and to my surprise my dear friend Patty showed up in the waiting room also. Friends and family, oh my they are priceless prayer warriors. And, this particular friend had been making intercession for me for years over the Fibromyalgia. Now there was this new physical interruption. Yes, it was bad news. There was a large tumor on my right ovary that appeared cancerous on the CAT scan image. As I sat there with the words Ovarian Cancer ringing in my ears, I went into mellow mode, humorously stating how my waistline will look so much better after the surgery. Then I looked into my husband's face and it was like nothing else I had ever seen. Gravity dissipated and we were hurled into the space of the unknown.

I was being arrested for misconduct in assuming my expanded stomach was associated with Fibromyalgia. What a shocking verdict I was given at that moment. For days I thought of my husband, my children, my grandson, and my whole family. I even began to label things in my house with their names so if I did die my husband would know which things went to whom. But then I began to pray.

Yes, but for prayer! Prayer and faith began to settle into my circumference and I was suddenly back in my happy bubble with Jesus. I had a real breakthrough that was not even logical. Those are the miracles that God can establish within us to break away the fear. So many people began to pray for me and I truly believe there was an army of Warriors circling around me. The prison I had found myself within was suddenly no more. The bars were open and I was released completely. No more labeling things as I choose to embrace each new day with the efficient grace that the Holy Spirit will give. Though I had a large bump in my road, I am not alone and I am not shaking in fear that the wicked witch is sending those nasty flying monkeys to attack me.

Nope, I click my heels and go home to the Father of Lights who surrounds me with a supernatural expression of his love. I am free.

The end of this story is; yes it was stage one cancer but isolated to only the ovarian cyst, which weighed a whopping 21 pounds. They removed it along with everything else I did not need. I am sure people wonder why it took me so long to go to a doctor. Well in part, Fibro fog, constant pain and an unhealthy dose of denial. Because I am over weight, I considered I was just gaining more weight. I am thankful God and logic woke me up that this wasn't normal at all.

So my story must awaken you all to be diligent, to talk with your doctor when any new concern breaks through the fog. Do not hesitate to fight for your freedom with knowledge, wisdom, and understanding. Be on your guard and stay awake in your pursuit for the fullest expression of abundant life.

CHAPTER 12

BEWARE OF MISCONCEPTIONS ABOUT ILLNESS AND LIMITED FINANCES IN SPIRITUAL INSTITUTIONS

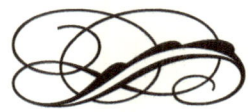

Even those religious communities that are supposed to help people can sometimes be a problem. Beware of what your religious community conveys to you in regards to health and finances. Now being a Christian, I can really only speak from my experience, but it is an experience worth sharing.

Now, I pretty much know my bible and after being a Christian for 30 years, when a part of the scriptures are presented in a manner that I do not agree with, I no longer freak out and go running from the church. But, if someone is new to the faith and scripture is falsely presented or just accidently presented in a manner that is not quite clear or accurate, it can crush someone and just add to the despair they already live with. For example, a few weeks ago I attended a church that I know is pretty solid and sound in doctrine. However, on this Sunday a guest speaker talked about the will of God for our lives. He stated that God's will is for all of us to be healed and to prosper financially. Well, that is what the bible states. I believe that this is God's perfect will for us. However, I also believe that given that we are in a fallen world, this is just not always the case; although, I believe we should continue to strive for it. So, while I am in agreement with the content, the presentation and elaboration on this doctrine was way off and potentially harmful to those who heard it. Let me explain in more detail.

While presenting this doctrine, the speaker stated that we were a poor witness to God if we were sick or poor and that we were really no use to God in this state. Now mind you, I was sitting there having fought chronic illness for 30 years and unfortunately broke.   Furthermore, I was doing everything possible to make both situations better. And I believe that I was seeking God's will. Now, if I did not understand that perhaps this speaker just presented it in a way that it sounded wrong or that maybe I misunderstood him, my heart would have been broken and I may never have gone back to church. I may have felt that perhaps God did not love me. But I know better. I know that God love's everyone of us no matter what condition we are in physically or financially. It simply does not matter to God. And, even during my worst years of being ill, I could still pray for others and often had others sit at my bedside while I helped them navigate some issue in their life. They trusted me because of my faith.

Now this isn't to say that we should accept whatever illness we are struggling with or financial lack, absolutely not. We should continue to seek healing by staying in the Word, looking at our lifestyle, and examining our thoughts and emotions. Perhaps by doing so, we will find ways to get better physically, emotionally, spiritually, and financially. It should be an ongoing journey. But when an illness does not leave or when finances just don't seem to get better, we can rely on a good and merciful God and know we are still loved and that our lives still matter. We can edify God by how we handle our situations in life, even when they don't seem to be changing. However, I am an eternal optimist and believe that God will answer our prayers and meet our needs in His time and in His way. Giving up is never an option.

Another piece to this teaching that really bothered me was when the preacher stated that people asking for help also did not make God look good. I was nearly floored. Now I do know some people that always have their hand out and continually ask for help and it doesn't look good. People tend to move away from them. But, it is ok to need help and to ask for help when you really need it. So many people suffer unnecessarily when there is help out there, both in social services and in the church.

Bottom line, in a healthy Christian Church, you should never be afraid of approaching the alter, and or an elder in the church, for prayer about anything, fearing you will be judged. You cannot be helped if you don't ask and church should be a safe place. At the same time, try to remember that a church is filled with imperfect people, so mistakes and misunderstandings can happen.

So if you are ever in a position where someone in spiritual authority speaks in a manner that you find makes light of what you feel and are experiencing in life, try to let it go. If you feel that talking to someone with some authority about it would help, do so in a non-confrontational manner. Remember, people are not perfect, but God is.

Diana Speaks:
There is a grace walk that a loving God has ordained and constituted for us to travel upon. That road is a journey in which we are never alone. We do not need to see what is ahead, we only need to see His face and the love that has become not only His pleasure, but our as well. The world around us can be seen through His lens and clarity can be a sweet release. If there is a Fibro fog, then it has no power in the unseen world. We can choose to release the physical obstacles into God's loving arms, or we can be policed by an illness that can feel criminal to say the least.

Most people have challenges in their lives that they need help with, need friendship and fellowship, and even spiritual guidance to get through. We can get help from a church, and we can give help, which in itself has a healing effect upon the giver and those who receive. Isn't that what Jesus did on the cross while enduring His greatest physical, emotional, and spiritual challenge. He gave love unto His last breath and we too can take that beautiful sacrifice into our own lives.

Like in any grouping of people, there can be one person, or more, who misunderstands the premise of grace and adds some legalized statements that can affix blame. Such as, you are not being healed because you lack faith or there is something wrong with you spiritually that is blocking Gods healing touch. I have heard that also; and, yes it bothered me a lot. It suggests that there was something I wasn't doing that I should do in order to get healed. You know what; I have not required God to heal me in order to find joy. I find joy and peace walking with God, period. I can get alone with Jesus and feel His presence while looking into His face of grace. We are not defined by an illness, we are created in the image of God and when this life is over and we exchange this body with a new one, we will never be in distress again. We shall never again cry out in pain or be attached to the chains of Fibromyalgia. I shall be free and while I wait, I shall gaze into the Master's face and cherish this journey I am now on.

I am healed and whole in Jesus name; and I do not have to see it in the physical realm. I can see it through His promise, for He is the keeper of my dreams and of my future in a place where there is perfect peace. The Lord truly is my Shepherd in this life and into the next. And so I follow the pathway that leads to green pastures. There I rest, and while I wait, I turn my eyes upon Jesus, look full in His wonderful face, and the things of earth will grow strangely dim in the light of his glory and grace. Amen

CHAPTER 13

ADAPTING TO A NEW WAY OF LIVING

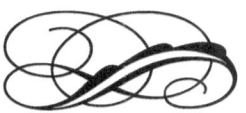

So now you get the picture, at least I hope you do. The question is how does one live with this illness and find enjoyment and fulfillment in life. I realize that not everyone shares my Christian faith, but everyone needs to find what will help get them through the dark times. Essential is to have someone to talk to. Fibromyalgia, like many chronic diseases, is a lonely walk. Having someone to talk to helps validate that you are not alone, or for that matter, that you are not losing your mind. My personal relationship with Jesus is my life savior. I may not have made it this far if it had not been for that. You see, when I got sick I did not have anyone to talk to. My friends and family always thought I had it all together, that I was strong. And I was, but even strong people need help. My family simply did not express their feelings and my father just thought since I was divorced, "that I made my bed so I should lay in it". So, where did I have to go when my life fell apart? The sad truth is I did not have anyone to turn to except my sister and one brother who I did not want to burden with my struggles. You see, I came from a family whose members were very successful and then there was me, in my mind, the loser because I could no longer function to my full capacity. So, I turned to God and He stepped in. I wish I could say it was easy and that everything got better all at once, but it didn't. It was a long, sometimes grueling walk. It still is. But I have found ways to cope, even to have fun. Most of all, I have found some peace and hope. I can't begin to tell you all the miracles that have happened in my life that can only be accredited to ongoing prayer and reliance on God. I know that many look at my life and see only the struggles; they don't see all the answered prayer. But that is a different book for a different time. This one was to help educate those with loved ones who suffer with Fibromyalgia and perhaps another "invisible illness" to better understand what is going on in their lives so they can better support them. And, for those who are struggling with Fibromyalgia, this book was to validate their suffering. No, you aren't crazy, it is an insidious disease.

That said; let's quickly look at just how someone can support a person with Fibromyalgia, or perhaps, a different chronic illness.

1. Never tell someone with Fibromyalgia that they are lazy or call them hypochondriacs. Yes support them in trying new things and in helping them move forward, but let it be at their own pace.

2. Don't get angry when someone with Fibromyalgia cancels an event with you. They probably just can't do it. However, you might want to look at ways they could make the event with some accommodations. For example, I once went away with three of my friends overnight to the beach. The next day they were going to walk around the ocean shore and I knew I could not. So, I brought along some blankets and while they were walking, I wrapped myself up in a blanket and lied on the beach, in the glorious sun. We all enjoyed the day. They were ok with me staying on the beach. That made it comfortable for me to go with them. Other times when I know that a lot of walking is part of an event, I plan ahead by bringing a book and finding a comfortable place to rest while others go ahead. The key is to talk about it and find ways that someone with limited movement can join in.

3. Recognize that someone on a fixed income like Social Security Disability has very limited resources. If you want them to participate in an event that costs money, be prepared for them to turn you down. Don't make them feel bad about not having the money. It is an awful feeling to be without money. If you have the money, offer to pay their way. Let them know that you are doing so because you want their company, not because you "pity" them.

4. Keep an eye on your loved one when you know they are going through a flare-up. They can become depressed and even suicidal. Let them know that they are not alone. Perhaps suggest they get out of the house and do something very low keyed, like going to a movie. Or, suggest you bring

a movie to them. If you think they are falling into a deep depression, get them to talk about it briefly and suggest they talk so someone, a therapist or someone at the church, if they go to one, that can pray for them.

5. If they are believers, and perhaps even if they are not, offer to bring them to church, to hear the healing word of God. If they are comfortable with it, get some people to pray for them. If not, put them on a prayer chain. Never underestimate the power of prayer and the power of the word of God.

6. Make sure they have the essentials to live with. Many people with Fibromyalgia and other chronic illness don't make enough money to live one. Casually note if they have food in the house and listen carefully to see if they might be behind on any major bill like rent, utilities, or even a car repair. If you find a need, see if you can help out personally, through the church, or through a social service agency. I know that several of my family members have noted my needs at times and found ways to put money in my hands. Even my father once paid off a charge I had run up that was all car repairs. They never made me feel less than because I was poor. Yup, I was poor. You are no less a person if you are poor. It is just an unfortunate economic state.

7. Finally, someone with Fibromyalgia needs empathy, not sympathy or pity. They need hugs, a kind word, and validation that they are ok even with a chronic illness. I remember once I was having a bad day and I told my brother

what a failure I felt like, not being able to work or take care of my children properly. His response was that he did not see me as a failure but rather as a courageous young woman who faced many trials and obstacles in her life. I cannot tell you how that one statement has gotten me through some tough times with my sanity intact.

People who suffer with Fibromyalgia need to know that God loves them just the way they are and that they can still be useful, functioning human beings, just in a different way. They need to be supported not tolerated. They need honestly not avoidance. And really, come on Christians; don't make the person with the chronic illness feel bad because God hasn't healed them. His ways our not our ways and we don't know what His plan is. Should you keep seeking healing and praying for that person's healing, by all means yes. But don't try to second-guess God, just continue to help the person keep seeking God and leave the rest to him.

So, now let's quickly review and look at ways to help one cope with Fibromyalgia actually live their life with purpose and enjoyment.

1.   Get a doctor who understands the illness you are living with. For me at first it was a doctor who understood CFS and since then, Fibromyalgia. You can't imagine, or maybe you can, how important it is to be able to walk into your doctor's office and say, "I feel like I am dying" and they get it. They don't think you are crazy or being dramatic. They get that this illness sucks the life out of you at times. It is

about empathy and validation. They also know what tests to take and what drugs may help. It is essential to have a doctor that understands this illness.

2. Don't be afraid to try medications, just be very careful. Like I mentioned, I try all new medications by taking 1/2 or 1/3 of the dose to start. Presently I take Doxepin, an anti-depressant that has been around for a long time. It is so very mild on my body and helps with depression and pain. I also take Klonopin, a benzodiazepine. It relaxes my muscles so the pain is not as intense; it relieves anxiety, and helps me focus during an episode of Fibo Fog. It is a lifeline for me. Many take a muscle relaxer instead, but I cannot as they make my heart race. Plus, Klonopin does more for me than just relax my muscles as I stated above. The danger is that Klonopin is highly addictive and you will develop some dependence on it if you take it for a long time. Well, I have taken for 20 years at the lowest dose and it still works. I probably do have some dependence on it, but the benefits far outweigh the risks. As I also mentioned, there are new drugs like Cymbalta, Lyrica, and other new drugs out there that help many. It is worth checking them out.

3. Work through the losses and emotional pain. Do not ignore it. Find a good therapist or someone you trust and you believe has wisdom to help you get through all the goodbyes and emotional struggles that this illness brings into your life. Ignoring them will block your ability to move past them and find a new, rewarding life for yourself. Learn to say your goodbyes. However, while you do need to talk about what

you are experiencing, you also need to be cautious to whom you talk to. I will explain why. First, many wonderful human beings just can't listen to it. It is not their calling. They can't handle it. Second, when you continually talk about it, you give your illness more power in your life. So choose wisely to whom you confide in. As I mentioned, I talk to my Christian Therapist and my friend Diana. I mention it to my other friends but only when necessary in making arrangements for an event or to voice a limitation. If you really think about it, how can you enjoy an activity when you are constantly talking about Fibromyalgia. Be very aware of how you handle this.

4. Find things you love to do so that you aren't thinking about having Fibromyalgia all the time. I love to read or go to the movies. Once engrossed in the movie or book, I think less about the pain or anything else that is bothering me. I also love to work and have found several part-time jobs that I can do. Guess what, when I am at work, doing things I enjoy, I don't notice the pain or fatigue as much. It works. Don't be afraid to try new things. It will be hit or miss at first, but you will find things that you enjoy.

5. I would love to say avoid stress, but that is just so hard to do. So what I will suggest is that you do try to avoid it when you are having a flare-up; and, when you can't, find ways to relieve it. Perhaps you can take a short walk, read a book, go home and turn off the phone, go to a movie, go to a prayer meeting, or do whatever you enjoy and makes you feel good.

6.   Try to maintain some type of exercise program. Now this is not an easy matter, so let's look at it for just a little bit. Many doctors just say to exercise. Is this good? No it is not. They don't know what they are talking about. Yes, we need to keep moving, but it really needs to be at your own, individual pace. And this takes time to discover. Let me try to explain. I started walking on the treadmill. At first I did 15 minutes at a slow pace, or walked outside at a slow pace. That was good for me. Now, after many years, I walk 30 minutes on the treadmill at a moderate pace, and even longer when outside. I love it. But, I always monitor my body. If it is in severe pain, I don't walk much. I may walk five or 10 minutes. I know to do too much will only set me back, not move me forward. I also use hand weights, only one pound, and only do 10 repetitions. However, when the Fibromyalgia is more active, I may only do two. I am careful not to overdo it, but I also always try to keep moving. However, there are times when the fatigue is so bad, I stay in bed for a day or two. So you see, exercise for someone with Fibromyalgia is a very personal thing. You need to find out what works for you.

7.   Finally, dig deep and find that part of you inside that gives you strength. As I said, mine is my personal relationship with Jesus. I can't put into words how this has saved and enhanced my life. You need to find that strength for yourself.

CHAPTER 14

WORKING THROUGH A FLARE-UP

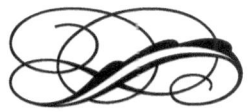

Now, I must confess, that it took me more than a year just to write this small book. You see, I went and got Lyme's disease just about a year ago and it went undetected for about 9 months. Lyme's disease just exacerbated the Fibromyalgia so it was difficult to even find the energy to write. But several months ago I did the protocol for the Lyme's and I have seen a huge difference already. I must state though, that as I was trying to figure out how to end this book, I began to go through a rather intense and painful flare-up and it dawned on me, that is how I would end the booklet. I would go through how I am dealing with this flare-up so I could pull together all my coping mechanisms to create a clearer picture on how I deal with these flare-ups. So here goes.

About two weeks ago I began to experience an increase in pain throughout my entire body. I also noticed that the fatigue and fibro fog was beginning to worsen. Well, I did not pay much attention to this and just kept pushing ahead. Now that was my first mistake. I know my body and I knew on some level that a flare-up was imminent. Well, after about a week or so of just "pushing through" I was really struggling with intense pain just getting worse. One afternoon after drying my hair I was standing in front of the mirror and just burst into tears. That is what I get for ignoring the pain. So, I got this bright idea that a long walk outside in the fresh air would help my mood and I proceeded to take this lengthy walk outside. By the time I got home, the pain in my legs was unbearable and I sat on the porch and cried some more. Finally, I got it, it was time to go into flare-up mode. Actually I might have prevented much of this pain if I had paid more attention to my body a week ago.

Let me tell you what I did that got me through this flare-up. Remember, it is different for each person. Most important is to acknowledge your need for going into flare-up mode. Then act quickly. First and foremost for me is to just slow down. I need to let go of any project that isn't urgently needed in the near future. For example, I needed to wash blankets and get my summer wardrobe ready, but none of this was urgent, so I let it all go. I only did what I had to do to keep my home in order and make sure I have clean clothes to wear. I also need to screen my phone calls and withdraw from any activity that is stressful, at least those that I am able to. In short, I have to become proactive in protecting my physical output and what I allow into my environment.

For me, slowing down and limiting my physical output

is difficult. I don't want to admit that I simply cannot keep up with my usual routine, it feels like defeat. But, I need to do that or I will just intensify the flare-up. So during a flare-up, I find that I have to walk slower and shorter distances. A few days after my crying jag, which is ok and often needed, I went to a beautiful shrine and walked slowly around its peaceful grounds. Being outside surrounded by the diverse and beautiful trees under a clear blue sky did wonders for my mood and walking, albeit limited and slow, made me feel like I was still exercising my body. After the shrine, I went with some friends to our favorite summer time restaurant and got a child's size frozen yogurt, raspberry chocolate chunk. Now, I got a child's size to honor my goal cf losing some weight. But, boy did I enjoy it. A few days later I went to a matinee movie and just sat back and enjoyed. I went to a matinee because the prices are much less than other times. When I plan activities, I always do so taking into consideration my budget, emotional, physical, and dietary limitations. During this flare-up I have also watched some movies on television and made it a point to take some long, hot baths, which help me a lot with pain control. I hope you are getting a general idea of ways you cannot just survive but find enjoyment during a flare-up.

Now sometime during this flare-up when I was feeling tired, worn out, and just plain overwhelmed, it just so happened that I was listening to Joyce Meyers, a Christian Teacher, when I heard her say the word "rest". She had spoken this word in the context of the bible scripture "Come to me, all you who are weary and burdened, and I will give you rest. Take my yoke upon you and learn from me, for I am gentle and humble in heart, and you will find rest for your souls." – Matthew 11:28-29. The entire scripture spoke to me but the word "rest" specifically resonated with me. So I sat on my coach, turned off all environmental sounds like the television and my phone, got comfortable, closed my eyes, and just let the silence permeate my body. For someone with Fibromyalgia, this complete silence and the rest that it brings our bodies is so soothing. For me, I take it a step further. While in this silent mode I pray. I purposely take anything that is causing me concern or stress and I hand them to God. I then quiet my mind and just focus on God, His mercy and love. He meets me here, in this silence. I can't explain just how I know, but I can often physically feel it. I just get this sense of well being, of being loved and cared for. As a Christian, I have come to understand that it is the Holy Spirit ministering to me in my time of need. I am not sure I could survive as well as I do without Him, the Holy Spirit. These moments remind me that God is in control and that if I let Him, He will meet my every need.

Diana Speaks:

"Never underestimate how wonderful you are, and please don't ever hesitate to shine out like a star. Not just a small and twinkling star that one can barely see, but a strong and bold and beaming light to guide the ships at sea.

Be strong in your convictions do not waver from the truth; ask of God for wisdom while you are in your youth. Ask of Him for knowledge and understanding too, of how to guide great ships at sea just by being you."

This is a verse from a poem my mother wrote for me as she inspired me to help those who are suffering with illness. As I watched her while I was growing up it was clear to me that my mother was certainly a strong and bold and beaming light, even in her weakest hours while suffering with this invisible illness. Her inspiration to help and to serve others came from the example of Jesus Himself.

My mom was taught about Jesus as a little girl by her mother, as I too was by mine. To know and be known by the Maker of the stars is in itself the greatest gift of all. My moms last words on this earth were to her Lord and Savior, even in the silent place of suffering He was there leading her into heaven where He would be her eternal cure.

I would like to finish my section of this book with the words of Jesus that have always brought me so much comfort. He is my resting place, as I cling to all His promises. There may be pain and suffering on this earth, but there is a place rich with life that never fades.

"Let not your heart be troubled: ye believe in God, believe also in me. In my Father's house are many mansions: if it were not so, I would have told you. I go to prepare a place for you. And if I go and prepare a place for you, I will come again, and receive you unto myself; that where I am, there ye may be also". John 14, 1-3 KJV

CHAPTER 15

LIFE CAN STILL BE GOOD

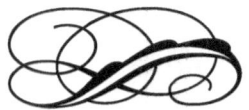

I am glad to report that as I conclude this book, the flare-up has ended. It lasted for about two weeks. Now I can walk outside again, dance just a little, and move about with much less pain. But, the flare-up didn't really end until I became proactive and paid attention to my body. I plan on enjoying every minute of not being in a flare-up. It is important to embrace the good times. And please, try to remember, you can live a life of meaning and joy even with Fibromyalgia or any other chronic Illness. You just have to be proactive. And, for those of you with Fibromyalgia, when you are struggling with a flare-up, try to remember, it won't last forever. And always, always, remember to keep close to your doctor, to try new treatments when they are suggested and your gut guides you in that direction, and be open minded to any suggestions that might help you better cope with the tough times. You can do it and you can find peace and joy in your life.

In closing, when I first began this journey with Fibromyalgia, this Bible verse jumped out at me and I have held onto the hope it represents now for 30 years. Meditating on it has often gotten me through some tough times. So, I want to share it with you.

He gives strength to the weary and increases the power of the weak. Even youths grow tired and weary, and young men stumble and fall; but those who hope in the Lord will renew their strength. They will soar on wings like eagles; they will run and not grow weary, they will walk and not faint. Isaiah 40:29-31 NIV

God Bless!